S0-ABB-066

On Being a Doctor 2

On Being a Doctor 2

Voices of Physicians and Patients

EDITED BY

MICHAEL A. LaCOMBE, MD

AMERICAN COLLEGE OF PHYSICIANS
PHILADELPHIA, PENNSYLVANIA

A|C|P

Manager, Books Publishing: David Myers
Administrator, Books Publishing: Diane M. McCabe
Production Supervisor: Allan S. Kleinberg
Production Editor: Victoria Hoenigke
Editorial Assistant: Alicia Dillihay
Designer: Kate Nichols

All selections in this book originally appeared in *Annals of Internal Medicine*, published by the American College of Physicians–American Society of Internal Medicine.

Composition by Fulcrum Data Services.
Printing/binding by R.R. Donnelley.
Printed in the United States of America.

American College of Physicians (ACP) became an imprint of the American College of Physicians–American Society of Internal Medicine in July 1998.

American College of Physicians–American Society of Internal Medicine
190 N. Independence Mall West
Philadelphia, PA 19106-1572

Library of Congress Cataloging in Publication Data

On being a doctor 2: voices of physicians and patients/edited by
Michael A. LaCombe.
p. cm.
ISBN 0-943126-82-7
1. Medicine Miscellanea. 2. Physicians' writings, American.
I. LaCombe, Michael A., 1942– . II. Title: On being a doctor two.
III. Title: On being a doctor 2.
R118.6.052 1999
610.69'52—dc21 99-40565
CIP

For a catalogue of publications available from ACP–ASIM, contact:
Customer Service Center
American College of Physicians–American Society of Internal Medicine
190 N. Independence Mall West
Philadelphia, PA 19106-1572
215-351-2600
800-523-1546, ext. 2600

00 01 02 03 04 / 9 8 7 6 5 4 3 2 1

Preface

Why You Should Read This Book

Why is *On Being a Doctor 2* unique? No other single book combines the experiences of being a doctor with those of being a patient, both expressed in exceptional prose and in the finest of poetry.

But more than that, if you are a physician and have lost a patient, or have been sued, or have suffered the frustrations of teaching in academia, or of caring for patients in present-day high-tech America, or if in the throes of managed care you remember the "good old days" of American medicine and wonder if they really were better days for us physicians, then be assured that someone has been there before you, has written about the experience, and that it is to be found among these pages. If you have faced the special challenges of being a woman in medicine or of bringing "first-world" medical knowledge to a third-world environment, you can compare your experiences with those of the physician-authors.

If you are or have been a patient, and have been pushed through the maze of bureaucracy that the medical system can be, or have profited from the miracles that modern medicine can bring, you will find patients, some physicians themselves, who have written with honesty and clarity about those same trials and triumphs.

If you belong to the large group of physicians who wish they read more often, and more about the human side of medicine, and who wish they could learn to appreciate good poetry and prose while at the same time wondering what it is that constitutes fine writing, you will find stories, essays, and poems to encourage your reading and sharpen your critical faculties.

Herein are the best recent pieces from the On Being a Doctor, On Being a Patient, and Ad Libitum sections of *Annals of Internal*

Medicine, selections that have undergone intense scrutiny by the editors and careful consideration by an independent board of reviewers. This compilation is largely of my own choosing; all have appeared since *On Being a Doctor*, the first collection of *Annals* pieces, was published in late 1994.

These three sections of *Annals* are very popular. The acceptance rate for submissions has remained about 15% for the past eight years. The rates of submission for the sections—about 12 to 15 manuscripts per month for On Being a Doctor, about 4 per month for On Being a Patient, and about 20 to 25 poems per month for Ad Libitum—attest to that popularity.

For some (admittedly biased) guidance through these pages, read the introductory essays for each of the three sections first.

Don't miss the poetry quiz. Which three poems do you think were award winners?

Above all, enjoy.

Michael A. LaCombe, MD
Harrison, Maine

Acknowledgments

To Frank Davidoff, Chris Laine, and David Goldmann, for their editorial direction, with special appreciation to F.D. for his innovation, *On Being A Patient*;

To Mary Beth Schaeffer and Caron Bell, for never losing a manuscript and for keeping us all on schedule;

And to David Myers, Diane McCabe, and Alicia Dillihay of the College's Books Division, for making this book possible,

Thank you!

Contents

Section I On Being a Doctor

Section II On Being a Patient

Section III Ad Libitum

CONTENTS

Section I

On Being a Doctor

Editorial guidelines for the "On Being a Doctor" section of the *Annals of Internal Medicine* ask for "short essays on illuminating experiences in practice" with a limit of 1500 words. (If it can't be said in 1500 words, it probably can't be said.) Both fiction and nonfiction are welcome. We, the editors, do not label any particular piece as "fiction" or "nonfiction," although we are frequently asked by readers whether a particular piece is "true." To some this matters; to others it does not, every piece in some measure being "true."

Having said that, allow me to label a few of the pieces reprinted here. Klein's *The Prison Patient* (page 54) was the most controversial, having generated no small amount of debate. It is fiction. Its ethical point—whether and how a physician may use his power over a patient for the common good—is "true." And perhaps more common an occurrence than we would like to admit. Costigan's *Trying To Let Go* (page 102) could only be nonfiction. It would take a very gifted writer indeed to convey in a fictional piece the pain and honesty portrayed here.

We are often asked by potential contributors: How does a manuscript make it into the pages of *Annals*? There are several ways:

- By the sheer force of good writing, as in Fitzgerald's *Curiosity* (page 5) and Van Peenen's *Marrying Medicine* (page 133).
- Through conveying brilliantly the magic that is medicine, as in Fournier's *The Gram Stain* (page 23) and Druss's *The Magic White Coat* (page 113).
- Through the clever use of humor, perhaps the toughest row to hoe in writing, demanding both sensitivity and a certain degree of self-effacement—see Casano's *Reimbursement over the Atlantic* (page 31) and Gensheimer's *The Making of a Public Health Physician* (page 92).
- By the compelling portrayal of ethical tension (Klein's *The Knight of Faith,* page 173) or the masterful use of mood, metaphor, and tone (Durso's wonderful *The Season's End*, page 16).
- Through the skillful narration of extraordinary encounters (Grubb's *Awakening,* page 13) or experiences (Rogal's *Brignole,* page 117).
- And, mostly, by relating common experiences in medicine in an exceptionally eloquent manner (McMurray's *Doctor's Daughter,* page 63, and her *Heartsick,* page 80).

Do editors have favorites? Yes, sometimes. My favorite in this section is *The Gram Stain.* But then, I'm from the old school!

Michael A. LaCombe

Curiosity

FAITH T. FITZGERALD, MD

About 15 years ago, when I was dean of students at the University of California, Davis, School of Medicine, yet another of the periodic paroxysms of "holism" in medicine occurred. Several importunate politicians called to tell me that, in their opinion—which presumably reflected that of their constituents—medical students, by selection or by their isolation by the medical curriculum, were insensitive, mechanistic, technocratic, inhumane brutes. The solution, these politicians insisted, was the intercalation of humanities courses into an already crowded curriculum.

I had several concerns about this. The first was that the addition of required courses in literature, drama, sociology, music, and art might actually limit students' opportunities to read, go to the theater, be with friends and family, and attend a symphony or museum. Even if one argues that students would not have done these things anyway—possessed as they were by the intricacies of glucose metabolism—the addition of these courses would cut down on contemplative time, volunteerism in free clinics, hobbies, and sleep. Second, I wondered what evidence supported the idea that being well versed in the humanities made one more humane. I was encouraged in my skepticism by the knowledge that perhaps the most broadly educated of physicians at the beginning of this century practiced in Germany. Moreover, I could not understand why science—a most human pursuit, the exercise of which is one of the defining characteristics of our species—should make students "inhumane." I decided to do a "scientific" study of the effects of humanities courses on humaneness in medical students.

Several colleagues and I read more than 10 years' worth of the subjective descriptions of performance of third- and fourth-year medical students on their clinical clerkships. We looked for adjectives suggesting humane behavior: "caring," "warm," "concerned," "good with patients and families." Each of these descriptors got "nice" points. Words like "callous," "abrupt," and "arrogant" got subtraction points. Then we compared "nice" points to the total number of units taken in the humanities in the student's premedical career.

What a shock: We found a direct correlation. I still thought it did not make sense. These were adults, after all. Was fundamental character, which is usually well formed by adolescence, changed by a class? I did what confused scientists have done for centuries to nonconforming data: I reanalyzed them. This time I ran a correlation between "nice" points and premedical units taken in science. Surprise again! Another direct correlation. Those students who had taken the most units in science had the highest number of "nice" points. In fact, in this idiot-driven experiment, "niceness" correlated directly with the total number of course units taken, regardless of the category.

What did it all mean? I did not know, but I wondered: What is kindness, as perceived by patients? Perhaps it is curiosity: "How are you? Who are you? How can I help you? Tell me more. Isn't that interesting?" And patients say, "He asked me a lot of questions"; "She really seemed to care about what was going on with me." Is curiosity the same, in some cases, as caring?

Curiosity is the urge to investigate, to discover. It can be seen in all small mammals; just watch a kitten explore a paper bag. Evidently, although curiosity can be dangerous ("What's down this dark hole, I wonder? What does this bright pill taste like? What's the funny-looking black animal with the white stripe down its back?"), it also has a redemptive adaptive function that exceeds the risks. Otherwise, puppies and small children would be wiped out. Curiosity is how we learn about our world.

Dr. Erich Loewy, in an unpublished paper, points out that curiosity, this primal "wonderment" that stimulates exploration, engages both imagination (conceiving the alternative explanations of new phenomena) and intelligence (mapping out the best way to determine which explanation is likeliest). Both imagination and intelligence are integral to humanities, science, and the synthesis of the two, which is clinical medicine. Rather than stating that the study of humanities makes one humane, I propose that humane people are curious and therefore choose to explore the humanities as well as the sciences.

An endowed lectureship at my medical school allows us to invite Nobel Prize-winning scientists to visit and lecture for several days. What impressed me most about my conversations with these luminaries was the extraordinarily broad range of their interests, their enthusiasm, and their thought patterns. One thinks science has a sequential and controlled pattern of logical ideas, firmly grounded in antecedent principles and constantly cleansed of intellectual debris by the abrasion of skepticism. Listening to Nobel laureates in medicine was revelatory. No linear thought here. They uninhibitedly threw forth multiple ideas in their observations, the connections between which were often invisible to me. As if the ideas were the small bright stones of a mosaic, forming many possible pictures, these scientists looked at them and rearranged them until they found a picture they liked. Dr. Baruch Blumberg, for example, explaining how he found the hepatitis B virus, told me stories of Australian aborigines, roof thatch, wombats, guitars, bedbugs, the Babylonian Talmud, and manned space flight. No doubt the disciplined thought of scientific proof came later.

The scientists seemed oblivious to intellectual constraints and unconcerned about being seen as naive or unknowledgeable. I suppose being a Nobel laureate means that one has little left to prove of one's adequacies as a thinker, but I have no doubt that these thought patterns preceded and were the reason for these people's Nobel-winning discoveries, not a consequence of the prize. Curiosity without constraint, no preconceived image to emulate, no need for the facade of competence, opening inquiry into any area that stimulated their interest—these qualities seemed common to them all.

In fact, the best clinical diagnostic thinking is more like the forming of a mosaic than linear thinking: It requires the physician to constantly alter diagnoses as each new piece of data enters the picture. One conceives constantly of many possible diagnoses, narrows down, reexpands, and generates an ever-evolving flux of ideas; the more information gained from patients, the better. For example, a 30-year-old woman with shortness of breath and fever (maybe a virus: pneumonia, of course) for 3 months (tuberculosis, multiple pulmonary emboli, lupus, sarcoidosis) recently returned from India (malaria, hepatic abscess, weird tropical diseases) where she was visiting her mother who was dying of breast cancer (anxiety; metastases from breast, ovarian, or colonic cancer; maybe she visited a guru and got toxic herbal medications), and so on.

What does curiosity have to do with the humanistic practice of medicine? Couldn't it just convert patients into objects of analysis? I believe that it is curiosity that converts strangers (the objects of analysis) into people we can empathize with. To participate in the feelings and ideas of one's patients—to empathize—one must be curious enough to know the patients: their characters, cultures, spiritual and physical responses, hopes, past, and social surrounds. Truly curious people go beyond science into art, history, literature, and language as part of the practice of medicine. Both the science and the art of medicine are advanced by curiosity.

One problem for medical students and physicians is that they must already have two things before engaging in uninhibited curiosity: a sense of competence (without which one tries to cultivate the appearance of competence, which generally means having more answers than questions) and time to think. The former is threatened by modern medical education and the latter by modern medical practice.

How is curiosity suppressed in medical students and physicians?

It is. I have discovered, in nonclinical settings, that students who, on the wards, seem totally without curiosity or culture—dolts, in short—were, in their private worlds, avid poets, artists, musicians, and craftspersons of exquisite skill, vitally interested in a wide range of topics. They just did not think it wise to let anyone know because they had received a message from housestaff, faculty, or peers that interest in anything other than purely biological medicine was inappropriate for a medical student.

Medical education itself suppresses the expression of curiosity, emphasizing examinable facts rather than more ineffable thought processes in order to provide reproducible experiences for students. It may even substitute virtual patients (case discussions, simulations, CD-ROMs, and syllabi) for real ones. Patients languish on the wards wondering who their physicians are while their physicians discuss abstract patients in small rooms or play diagnostic games on the computer. Acting as a preceptor to second-year students, I discovered to my dismay that they gave up a physical diagnosis session to study for the written examination in physical diagnosis. Does this make sense?

Efficiency, in which patients are seen as "work units," also suppresses curiosity. One senior resident once presented a patient in morning report and, as part of the physical examination, mentioned a scar in the patient's groin. When I asked how the scar had been acquired, she said, "He told me he was bitten by a snake there."

"How did that happen?" I asked.

"I don't know," she said.

How could that be? How could one not ask? The imagination runs riot with the possibilities of how this man got bitten by a snake in the groin. But the resident was too busy (or not curious enough) to ask!

The sacrosanctity of print and the ancient human belief that what is written is more true than what is said suppress curiosity. A third-year student presenting a patient to me at the bedside told me that the patient had had "BKA [below-knee amputation] times two." Standing there, I saw that the patient had legs. I asked the student, "Did you find legs on your physical examination?"

"Yes," he said.

"How then did he have bilateral below-the-knee amputations?" The student was confounded. He could not understand it. He was struck mute. He reached out and touched the legs: warm, hairy, clearly the patient's own and not prosthetics.

"I don't know," he said.

"What makes you think the patient had bilateral below-the-knee amputations?"

"It said so in the chart." We got the chart, and indeed, for this patient's past three admissions, "BKA times two" was listed under history. It was only after looking at the past five admissions that the transcriptionist's error became clear. The patient had been previously admitted twice for diabetic ketoacidosis—DKA. But once typed, BKA became enshrined chart lore and was repeated by every subsequent house officer as if it were true, even in the face of the evidence of their own senses.

Technology is wonderful and seductive but, when seen as more real than the person to whom it is applied, it may also suppress curiosity. When I was a house officer and installing one of the first right-heart catheters, the machine that showed intrapulmonic arterial pressures was enormous and was equipped with strain gauges rather than computer chips. Making it work was difficult. After the line was in, the attending, the nurse, and I tried desperately to adjust the machine to show the pulmonary arterial pressure waves. We could not get them. The line on the screen remained flat. We manipulated toggle switches and strain gauges for about 15 minutes. Nothing. Finally, I glanced at the patient: He was dead. We had been so engaged with the machine that we had missed this significant clinical event, which explained why the pulmonary arterial pressures were unobtainable. We assumed that the answer to the question lay in the machine and explored no further until it was too late.

What is the reward of curiosity? To the patient, it is the interest and physical propinquity of the physicians, which is therapeutic in and of itself. To the physician, curiosity leads not only to diagnoses but to great stories and memories, those irreplaceable "moments in medicine" that we all live for. When I was a young attending at San Francisco General Hospital, morning rounds usually consisted of briefly going over the 15 or 20 patients admitted to the team the night before and then concentrating on the "interesting" ones. I was righteous and was determined to teach the housestaff that there were no uninteresting patients, so I asked the resident to pick the dullest.

He chose an old woman admitted out of compassion because she had been evicted from her apartment and had nowhere else to go. She had no real medical history but was simply suffering from the depredations of antiquity and abandonment. I led the protesting group of housestaff to her bedside. She was monosyllabic in her responses and gave a history of no substantive content. Nothing, it seemed, had ever really happened to her. She had lived a singularly unexciting life as a hotel maid. She could not even (or would not) tell stories of famous people caught in her hotel in awkward situations. I was getting desperate; it did seem that this woman was truly uninteresting. Finally, I asked her how long she had lived in San Francisco.

"Years and years," she said.

Was she here for the earthquake?

No, she came after.

Where did she come from?

Ireland.

When did she come?

1912.

Had she ever been to a hospital before?

Once.

How did that happen?

Well, she had broken her arm.

How had she broken her arm?

A trunk fell on it.

A trunk?

Yes.

What kind of trunk?

A steamer trunk.

How did that happen?

The boat lurched.

The boat?

The boat that was carrying her to America.

Why did the boat lurch?

It hit the iceberg.

Oh! What was the name of the boat?

The *Titanic*.

She had been a steerage passenger on the *Titanic* when it hit the iceberg. She was injured, made it to the lifeboats, and was taken to a clinic on landing, where her broken arm was set. She now was no longer boring and immediately became an object of immense interest to the local newspapers and television stations—and the housestaff.

For whatever reason—economics, efficiency, increased demands on physicians for documentation, technology, or the separation of education from patient care—curiosity in physicians is at risk. I believe it is our duty, as those who now teach young physicians, to identify medical students with a gift for curiosity and take infinite pains not to suppress but to encourage that gift. Not only will patient care be enriched, but so will the lives of these physicians and the vigor of our art and science. Besides, it will be much more interesting.

Awakening

BLAIR P. GRUBB, MD

There were so many admissions that night that I had begun to lose count—and my temper. A seasoned intern, I had learned well the art of the quick, efficient work-up. Shortcutting had become a way of life. Morning was coming and, with it, my day off. All I wanted was to be done. My beeper sounded. I answered it. I heard the tired voice of my resident say, "Another hit, some 90-year-old Gomer with cancer." Swearing under my breath, I headed to the room. An elderly man sat quietly in his bed. Acting put upon, I abruptly launched into my programmed litany of questions, not really expecting much in the way of answers. To my surprise, his voice was clear and full and his answers were articulate and concise. In the midst of my memorized review of systems, I asked if he had ever lived or worked outside the country.

"Yes," he replied. "I lived in Europe for 7 years after the war." Surprised by his answer, I inquired if he had been a soldier there.

"No," he said. "I was a lawyer. I was one of the prosecuting attorneys at the Nuremberg trials." My pen hit the floor. I blinked.

"The Nuremberg trials?" He nodded, stating that he later remained in Europe to help rebuild the German legal system.

"Right," I thought to myself, "some old man's delusion." My

beeper went off twice. I finished the examination quickly, hurried off to morning sign-out, and handed over the beeper.

Officially free, I started out the door but suddenly paused, remembering the old man, his voice, his eyes. I walked over to the phone and called my brother, a law student, who was taking a course on legal history. I asked him if the man's name appeared in any of his books. After a few minutes, his voice returned.

"Actually, it says here that he was one of the prosecution's leading attorneys at the Nuremberg trials." I don't remember making my way back to his room, but I know I felt humbled, small, and insignificant. I knocked. When he bid me enter, I sat in the very seat I had occupied a short time before and quietly said, "Sir, if you would not mind, I am off duty now and would very much like to hear about Nuremberg and what you did there. And I apologize for having been so curt with you previously." He smiled, staring at me.

"No, I don't mind." Slowly, with great effort at times, he told me of the immense wreckage of Europe, the untold human suffering of the war. He spoke of the camps, those immense factories of death, the sight of the piles of bodies that made him retch. The trials, the bargaining, the punishments. He said that the war criminals themselves had been a sorry-looking bunch. Aside from the rude awakening of having lost the war, they could not quite understand the significance of the court's quiet and determined justice or of the prosecution's hard work and thorough attention to detail. The Nazis had never done things that way. So moved had he been by the suffering he encountered there that he had stayed on to help build a system of laws that would prevent such atrocities from happening again. Like a child I sat, silent, drinking in every word. This was history before me. Four hours passed. I thanked him and shook his hand, and went home to sleep.

The next morning began early, and as usual I was busy. It was late before I could return to see the old man. When I did, his room was empty. He had died during the night.

I walked outside into the evening air and caught the smell of the spring flowers. I thought of the man and felt despair mixed with joy.

Suddenly my life seemed richer and more meaningful, my patients more complex and mysterious than before. I realized that the beauty and horror of this world were mixed in a way that is sometimes beyond understanding. The man's effect on me did not end there. Despite the grueling call schedule, the overwhelming workload, and the emotional stress of internship, something had changed within me. I began to notice colors, shapes, and smells that added magic to everyday life. I learned that the gray-haired patients that I had once called "Gomers" were people with stories to tell and things to teach. After nearly two decades, I still look to that night, remember that man, and reflect on the chance and privilege we have to share in the lives of others, if only we take the time to listen.

The Season's End

SAMUEL C. DURSO, MD

Sometimes Ezra would kid about the future. "What'll happen when I'm gone?" he would ask with mock seriousness. "The fish and ducks will rest a lot easier."

We would both laugh, exchanging glances like friends playing poker, looking for a hint of change in the other's expression.

It had been a year since I met Ezra. I had become his student of sorts, following him all over the tidal marshes surrounding our hometown, Port Arthur, Texas. I was his doctor, too, and he couldn't help asking me often in his casual, by-the-way manner, "How am I doing, Doc?"

Using my doctor's eye, I would look at him and say, "Fine, Ezra! You feel fine, don't you?"

"Sure, man, I'm better than I ever was."

He looked tan and fit although I knew that his heart was large. I marveled, comparing him now with my mind's image of him the day I first met him, sitting on the edge of his hospital bed, wearing pajamas, a translucent oxygen tube looped over his face. That day, the opening day of duck season, a hunting companion had persuaded him to leave the marsh and come to my office. During the preceding weeks, he had often been short of breath, and that morning he was short of breath just standing in his blind. It did not take long to make the diagnosis. I sent him straight to the hospital.

In duck hunting circles around Port Arthur, Ezra was a legend. He was a champion duck caller, and good hunters respectfully conceded to him. "How did you learn duck calling, Ezra?" I asked while he was still seated on the hospital bed.

"Doc, I'll tell you something," he said, in an East Texas drawl that was peppered with Cajun. "I've made duck calling records—I'll give you one, if you want—but you can't really learn to call a duck the way I call them by listening to records. Everything I know about calling I learned from ducks. You can hear some people call a duck, and it sounds beautiful, like they was playing a musical instrument. They blow their caller like they was in a band, but the ducks just fly by. They don't even look down." He shook his head a little, as if telling something that was almost pathetic.

There was a story in his answer.

Meeting and knowing a master intrigued me. Even in my own field, I had met very few. Ezra was part of a rare group. He had a drive that kept him chasing one of nature's secrets. Like all masters, he had learned to apply himself patiently in order to understand something thoroughly. Something that looked mysterious to ordinary folk became a force under his control. He didn't work at his skill halfway, either. He learned it by sitting for hours, hidden in salt grass, watching and listening.

Ezra must have been looking for someone to teach even before he became ill. He was particular about who he would let around him, and he had not "brought someone up," as he put it later, for years. He didn't care to have someone slow him down, but he liked the way I listened and decided to take me as his partner. He knew I wanted to learn.

In the hospital, he said, "Doc, you're steering me right. I'm gonna stick to you like glue. You know what they say, 'Gotta dance with the one that brung you.' You ever been in the marsh?"

"Truth? No. Even raised here. I've never hunted it, been in it, or anything."

"Let me take you, Doc, and you take care of me."

"Sure. But you've gotta get stronger. Let's see how you do when you get home; you've gotta get back on your feet first."

"Aw, man, I'm gonna do what you say. You're the boss! Whatever you say. We can take it easy. Okay. One step at a time!" he said, his voice rising.

"Yeah, we'll see how you do once you're out of the hospital."

He was already planning ahead. "All right, I'm dancing with the one that brung me! Whew, boy!" he exclaimed, this time letting out a Cajun yelp. I couldn't believe his excitement. I hoped that I hadn't oversold him on his recovery. He had a weak heart, possibly a viral cardiomyopathy, and I had no idea how well he would do.

During the next year, he got back on his feet and then some. I even wondered sometimes if I had made the right diagnosis. There were times when I barely kept up with him. Tests confirmed that his heart was weak, but nothing could measure his will; it was the strongest I had ever encountered. He took his part of our partnership seriously, too, rousing me more mornings than I wanted so that I could be up with him before dawn, in the marsh, and back before rounds at the hospital. During that year, it seemed that every waking minute I wasn't in the office or in the hospital, I was in the salt marsh, learning as fast as I could absorb Ezra's lessons.

Still, all that time I was keeping an eye on him, too. I thought sometimes that I sensed in him a bit of fatigue, a little tiring in his fight. It was hard to say. He had a way of conserving energy and working things so that he could take a short break when he needed one. He didn't want me telling him to rest, but if I rested, he would. His competitive nature prevented him from showing any sign of slacking. If he caught me watching his breathing after he finished slogging a few hundred yards through ankle-deep mud, he countered by asking me, "You all right?"

"Sure, I'm all right, Ezra. This marsh's put me in good shape."

"It'll do it. It's the best thing for you, Doc."

One winter day, Ezra and I made a trip to the marsh for a late afternoon hunt. It was the last day of duck hunting season and a little over a year since I had met him. We were driving out to Los Patos, known as the "duck ranch," a piece of privately owned Gulf Coast marsh marked off by miles of barbed wire.

Ezra was driving his old green pickup, which had a salvaged camper over the bed. Leaning forward in his seat, both arms folded over the top of the steering wheel, he talked while I poured us a sip of coffee. He was in a good mood. He looked over with a kind of earnest expression, as if about to thank God for his good luck, and said, "Man, Doc, I've got it made in the shade, don't you think?" He didn't need a direct answer. "I mean, look at this. We're headed to Los Patos, the best duck hunting in the world. What else do I need? When this season is over, I can fish it or crab it to my heart's content. The owners don't care. All they want is for me to keep up the blinds and take 'em for hunts. What's easier than that?"

I had to nod. Of course, I was the luckiest person of all because I was stuck like glue to the best duck hunter in the world in the best marsh in the world.

We pulled up to the entrance of Los Patos. I got out of the truck's cabin to unlock the gate. With my back to the Gulf of Mexico, I swung the gate wide, holding it open for Ezra to drive through. The best part of opening the gate came with smelling air fresh with Gulf surf. To either side of the gate, I could see the effect of the gusting winds whipping over fields of salt grass, picking up the tangy scent of fermenting grass-straw. When I stepped off the road into the brackish salt marsh, I could easily appreciate the generative union between land and sea. What I missed on the highway from the truck's cabin could be seen closely by looking down at the tannic water between my boots. There, mosquito larvae and minnows fought out their existence. A sea of salt grass stretched far to the distant intercoastal canal. Los Patos was big, a wetland representative of the Gulf Coast plain, lying within the central flyway for ducks and geese migrating from Canada to Mexico and back. This was heaven for Ezra.

Today, he wanted to try something different. His idea was to walk as far as we could to an area where he could call down pintails that were wary of hunters this late in the season. He wanted to get there on foot; he was convinced that pintails were staying far away from the sight of airboats. It would be hard work. We pulled on waders and packed shells and coffee thermoses into green five-gallon buckets that Ezra had camouflaged by spraypainting them brown and black. Carrying shotguns and buckets, we took off in a new direction for the last afternoon hunt of the season.

Finding a spot of ground in front of a little open water, we put down our buckets and pulled salt grass up into a blind. We settled in, talking a little and scanning the sky overhead. Not much happened while we sipped coffee. Suddenly, Ezra crouched low, pointing to a thin line of ducks in the distance. They were barely visible to me; I could just make out the characteristic wing movement. Ezra said they were pintails. I still couldn't understand how he could tell pintails from mallards at that distance. They didn't seem to be in calling range, but he had two callers of his own making hanging from a string around his neck, and he put one to his mouth, opening with an incomparable, authentic call. The wind was blowing into our faces. At first, I couldn't see much response in the ducks. Ezra put a bigger effort into his caller.

"I'm gonna hit 'em with this, Doc." He put out a long distress call.

I didn't know if he could reach them. Then I saw their flight make a shift. The lead ducks picked up his call. Their flight changed with small jerks, as if in indecision. They turned tentatively toward us. Soon it was certain: He had locked them with his calls. At first, the ducks were a few thin streams of distant cirrus trails. Then the lead ducks turned toward our blind, and the trails coalesced. A boiling gray cloud of 100 ducks headed straight for us. In the process of coming closer, pintails in groups of 10 began dropping down. I knew that within seconds they would be whistling by our blind. I kept my head down, eyes turned on Ezra, waiting for that split second when he would look at me to signal, "Now!"

Instead, he whispered, "Aw, Doc, this is too easy." He shook his head as if he couldn't believe how pathetically easy it had been.

His words took me by surprise, but I knew I had heard him right. I eased back onto the overturned bucket I used for a seat. A sharp catch in my neck relaxed as I turned my head from Ezra. The ducks were landing with light splashes. I felt my heart beating in my ears. In seconds, only the hum of mosquitoes and the soft, undisturbed feeding chatter of the ducks surrounded us.

I looked back at Ezra. He, too, was uncoiled from his hunting crouch, sitting on his bucket, his worn Browning 12-gauge across his lap. He looked at the ducks and the marsh.

I studied my mentor out of the corner of my eye, and I looked at the ducks on the marsh, too. Ezra was a master duck hunter. The greenhead's tail feathers trimming the band of his dress Stetson were real enough. But this was another matter.

I thought over his comment. "This is too easy." It wasn't, of course. That was an ironic understatement; only his great effort had taken us to this point. But now I realized something else. Even as I had learned from him as my mentor and patient, I had not foreseen the possibility of this change. He had redefined himself, or maybe it would be more accurate to say that he had prepared himself. Perhaps the change occurred while he was conceding something to his illness. Perhaps not. I could only guess, but I suspected that minutes ago, having visited the pinnacle of his skill, he had seen an image of himself that looked small against the magnificent image of those ducks responding to his pleading call. This was his awakening experience, an integration of himself and his universe. Rather than struggling for another instant of mastery over nature, he instead stopped and sought simply to reflect on life. I never asked him, but he must have been willing to view himself, and be viewed, differently, as a person who was willing to relinquish mastery over life long enough to become part of a greater whole.

The afternoon sun shone in the pale winter sky. A cool Gulf Coast breeze fluttered over the marsh, occasionally touching down and wrinkling the water's smooth surface, erasing reflections of fast-moving clouds overhead. We sat there quietly, without regard for time, until for no reason except that known to the ducks, the pintails suddenly rose from the water, beating their wings, and, like one of the clouds overhead, pushed away.

Ezra grinned. We gathered up our buckets and shell boxes and left. We were through for the season.

The Gram Stain

ARTHUR M. FOURNIER, MD

The intern on my ward team presented her patient succinctly: "A 38-year-old man presents with a 1-week history of fever, pleuritic chest pain, and rust-tinged sputum. Chest x-ray shows a lobar infiltrate."

"Sounds like pneumonia," I offered. "What did you treat him with?"

"Timentin and gentamicin, one dose . . . He was in the hospital just a few weeks ago . . . We couldn't be sure what we were treating . . . ."

"Fever, pleuritic pain, rust-tinged sputum, lobar infiltrate—sounds like strep pneumonia to me. Penicillin is still a wonder drug against strep pneumonia, and it's so inexpensive. Why not do a Gram stain and be sure of what you're treating?"

My resident leaped to his intern's defense.

"Dr. Fournier, they don't let us do Gram stains any more. . . . It's against the law. . . . They throw us out of the micro lab." Sarcastically, he added, "They don't trust our judgment."

"Yeah, I know that law . . . CLIA [Clinical Laboratory Improvement Amendments]." I screwed up my face, trying to decide whether I should tell them what I really thought of these regulations. "No patient with pneumonia should be started on antibiotics without the physician first looking at a Gram stain."

"But Dr. Fournier, what can we do?"

"Civil disobedience!" My eyes grew wide, and the veins in my neck stuck out. "Follow me!"

I picked up a sputum specimen from the patient and an alcohol pledget from a crash cart. We left the emergency department and crossed a corridor to an unmarked door. I turned the handle. It was unlocked. I led the team into one of the old house officers' laboratories. Dust layered the counters, coating the microscope, the staining bottles, and the laboratory paraphernalia. Cobwebs stretched from the microscope's objectives to the stage mount.

"The Holy Grail," I whispered reverently. The housestaff stared at me as if I'd lost it.

I brushed away the cobwebs and cleaned the eyepiece and objectives with a scrap of lenspaper. I teased a specimen of thick, green sputum from the cup and spread it on a slide.

"How will you heat-fix it, Dr. Fournier? They've shut off the gas on the Bunsen burner."

I was too excited to answer. I opened the alcohol pledget and twisted the foil so it could stand on end. I placed it in the sink, lit the exposed edge with a safety match, and watched nostalgically as the yellow flame with its blue center rose about 2 inches above the pledget.

"Behold the Boston City Hospital Bunsen burner," I pronounced. The team stared, transfixed like moths by the flame. After three passes through the flame, the slide was ready for staining. Crystal violet, Gram's iodine, acetone, and safranin. How many times had I repeated this litany? My thumb and index finger received first the purple and then the red stigmata.

"Once upon a time, we could tell which housestaff had been on call by whose fingers were stained," I said to no one in particular.

Then I entered yesteryear, that timeless world of purple and red, the bizarre denatured shapes of stained nuclei and cytoplasms. I could be an intern again. Once upon a time, every patient that was admitted to the hospital had peripheral smears and microscopic urinalyses examined by an admitting intern. Any possibly infected body fluid was always Gram-stained. It was part of the physical exam. Now, scanning past the squamous cells, looking for good sputum, I went in for a closer look.

"There! The enemy!" I exclaimed to the third-year student at my shoulder. "Look, right in the poly in the center of the field. . . those pairs of blue dots with the haloes around them. . . strep pneumonia. . . ."

The young student took off her glasses and squinted as she adjusted the fine focus. She paused.

"Cool!"

Caring for Strangers

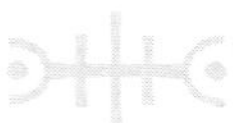

MICHAEL A. LaCOMBE, MD

The quiet young girl with thick eyebrows arching over blue eyes sat quietly, waiting for her chin to be sewn, and took it all in. The room was nearly full. Most of the people waiting with her were familiar to her, seemed to know her, glanced from her to her mother and formed the unspoken gossip with their eyes. This was life in a small town. She avoided their stares much as she suppressed the pain of her chin. Looking through the door, she saw the starched white nurses waiting on the doctor. She didn't ever want to wait on anybody. She wanted to be waited on. The doctor had something in his right hand, brought it down to a bare leg, then away, then down and away again. The girl caught the pungency of iodine, the steel-sharp scent of alcohol. There were old magazines she didn't want to read and a chart of fruits and vegetables on the wall. She was bored. She was tired. She was hurting.

"Next," said the skinny nurse, and the young girl followed her mother into the next room. She sat on the table, tried to cover the rip in the knee of her jeans with a hand, and looked around.

"How old are you, honey?" asked the older nurse with the glasses on a chain. "Has she had her shots?" she asked the girl's mother.

"Nine," said the girl.

"Yes," said her mother. "They're up to date."

"Dee-Pee-Tee?"

"Just last year, in school," answered her mother.

Laughter shot from the adjacent examining room, then shuffling, a clinking of metal on glass, and the doctor breezed in. He was tall, young, happy-looking. He probably had kids of his own.

"My God," he said, "what beautiful eyes! And your eyebrows, young lady. . . ."

"She takes after her father," said the girl's mother. "Those are his bushy black eyebrows." Privately, the girl loathed her eyebrows. She would pluck them as soon as she got home to her room.

"Yes," said the surgeon, "oh yes, I see. . . ."

He knows about the divorce, thought the young girl. Everybody in town knows about the divorce.

"It's down to bone," said the surgeon to no one in particular. "Pretty bad cut, actually. It'll take some time . . . three layers. June," he said, lifting his head to the older nurse and nodding toward the waiting room, "see if Bob can come down and help with them."

The shot stung severely, and then her chin went numb. Stitching the wound took more than an hour—she was a pretty girl, after all, and the surgeon, skilled enough in plastics, took his time with her. Through the drape covering her face, the young girl answered with staccato yeses and noes the surgeon's questions about school, about play, about friends and pets and brothers and sisters. But with the mind of a discontented, troubled 9-year-old, she heard more than questions and felt far more than her simple answers. The surgeon's voice was not the harsh, abusive, slurred male voice to which she had been accustomed. This voice was kind and deep, holding gentleness rather. She felt touched by it and its caress, allowed herself to be soothed by it, permitted herself a small bit of hope and a fleeting arousal of what she would later call love.

"It's like Cassiopeia," said the surgeon. "You know, the constellation Cassiopeia. Your laceration, it's a sort of lazy W, like Cassiopeia." And it was in this way that his pet name for her came to be.

For the next 4 years, until puberty struck her like a hot shower, the young girl cherished that moment with the surgeon, frequented the hospital through any excuse to volunteer or visit, so she might happen upon him, to hear him call her Cass, to feel him touch the lazy W on her chin, and to bask in the attention of her secret, very part-time surrogate father.

But together with Chance's shifts and realignments, with Progress' seeming advance and sorry decline, 14 years more passed by. For the young girl, now a handsome young woman in hip-length white coat, stethoscope slung around neck, pockets jammed with note-cards, black book, pins, percussion hammer, and tuning fork, these were years of frenetic pace and postponement—years of endless study and ceaseless competition, of anatomy and melancholia, of friends who never were, of slices of nephrons stared at through exhausted eyes rather than slices of life consumed through eager lips. These were years of quick sex for its own sake rather than relationships for the hope of intimacy, and, for the young woman particularly, these were years of searching for other surrogate fathers. In the dust of memory mingled with tragedy of another kind, she had long since forgotten her surgeon of childhood. He had moved on to the City himself, a casualty of circumstance and life, and she had supplanted him with others—for one, with the cardiologist who had taught her physical diagnosis and who had taught her as well that a patient was merely a good case, demonstrated great clinical findings and little else, and that there were other great cases to be found rather than any story to be listened to. From this man she moved on to the senior resident who taught her how to take the history while examining the patient at the same time and, by so doing, minimize time spent with each hit. She slept with this resident as though it were part of the rotation, and while he worried about keeping it from his wife, she worried about The Match. It was all part of the hardening-up process, a part of this training of the physician of today. Legacy and tradition were never to tread upon her character.

She was always there, always on the wards, always to be seen, noticed, appreciated. When she wasn't on call, she'd read about the other students' admissions, deftly one-upping them the next morning on teaching rounds. This was how you got ahead. She quickly learned that the professors were human, most of them every bit male, and so learned to dress and comport herself with just the proper degree of seductiveness. In this huge new world of Medicine as Business, of patients as clients, and of doctors as providers, she too was a commodity, after all. And the bottom line for her, while not yet money, was clearly the top of the ladder.

The first years of residency she merely endured. There was little else one could do. When not serving up caths for the cardiologists, she was sorting through the stroked-out gomers, trash bags, and drunks in the emergency room. She had long since forgotten the quiet calm of the community hospital whose halls she had walked as a child. Now, this waiting room held druggies poised to infect her with HIV, alcoholics ready to vomit on her, and the swinging, lurching wildness of the crazed dirtballs whom she would punish in return with Foley and large-bore Levine.

The last residency year was better. She could glimpse the light at the end of the tunnel: the fellowship that would rescue her from this dark-alley existence and deliver her to the high-tech, pristine calm of the consultant. There was odd relief, too, in helping those poor bastards beneath her in training contend with what she had only too recently had to stomach herself, assisting them with last night's hits and today's drooling dispositions. She knew the ropes now, could teach them the short cuts, the quick paths around the crap of patient care. The attendings sympathized, of course. This was the medicine of today, the business of having to earn all of one's salary through patient care, make money for the department, and please the chief so he could be away. This was the mythical time of universal coverage in which indigents' costs were covered by seeing ever more patients faster and more efficiently. This was the time of the in-and-out, touch-the-shoulder race of bedside teaching rounds. It was the era of case presentation, with films on the viewing box, data on the blackboard, bagels and coffee on the conference table.

As a fellow, the young woman began again to be excited about medicine. Now one of the boys, she began to be treated like the men, except on that occasion when allowing herself to be treated like a woman might further her own career, all the while learning from the men of medicine how one gets by in a man's world. Medicine as a discipline became more focused, narrowed, manageable, her hours more reasonable, sleep coming more predictably and in greater quantities. "Cases" now were consults. Now she could be insulated by intern, resident, and attending from the dirtball and his obligatory rectal exam. Now she could think in terms of pre-excitation rather than palpitation, plaque formation rather than chest pain, and wires and devices, forgetting the tedium of a tiresome patient's fainting spells.

Oh, still the occasional consult might bring her too close to the patient and that hell of early residency. Even now she might be compelled to linger at the bedside while some goddamn student with whom she had been saddled to teach and who wouldn't take "it doesn't matter" for an answer searched for the diastolic sound. That there might ever be in these encounters with patient and student the chance of missed occasion never occurred to this young woman who had been once long ago a constellation of infinite possibility.

So it was this night. Once more she had been summoned to the maelstrom of the emergency ward. Yet again she leaned over this patient "found down," careful not to touch him, placed the bell of her stethoscope over precisely the right spot and handed the earpieces to the student to get this "teaching moment" done with, while this patient, swimming frantically to consciousness and blue with cyanosis, gasping from dyspnea, soaked wet with the work of breathing, stared at her even as she felt his stare and loathed and avoided it, peered at her disbelieving and caught the thick, black eyebrows that had become her signature, caught the cobalt blue of her eyes, hurried his gaze frantically to the lazy W of her chin, recalled his own surgical precision, and eased within himself, thinking,

"Cassiopeia. . . . Thank God. I am in good hands."

Reimbursement over the Atlantic

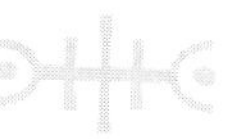

A. ANDREW CASANO, MD

Two unrelated issues came to mind as I reflected on a recent harrowing experience. One was the heated debate over the imbalance in financial reward between medical–surgical procedures and so-called cognitive activity or (forgive me) non-procedures. The second was the solid foundation of traditional Western medical education on which I was fortunate enough to capitalize.

It seems that in medicine we have developed a curriculum that is effective, even for those of us who only practice part-time and cannot be on the cutting edge of technology with its latest generation of cephalosporins. It is a credit to traditional medical education that when occasionally challenged by friends, family, and the few patients for whom I take responsibility, I can draw on the strong foundation of fundamentals available in every U.S. medical school. This method does not require enormous amounts of detail close at hand, but simply a logical sequence of steps to organize symptoms and signs, focus on a few potential organ systems, and then make a diagnosis. This leaves the obscure and the incurable for textbooks and keener minds.

Now, having said this, I must quickly admit that I do not have the same confidence when it comes to medical emergencies. I have willingly stepped aside for the eager emergency medical technicians in public places where my interim help as a physician was sought. Frankly, I was glad to yield as I barked a few officious platitudes so that all present might have no doubt as to who was in charge. A once-proud knight in white cotton pants who could cannulate any orifice in an emergency, I now secretly hope none of my middle-aged golf partners suffer a medical catastrophe over a 2-foot putt.

This introduction will explain why I was less than eager to respond when an announcement requesting a physician came over the intercom 1 hour into my transatlantic flight to Berlin and Warsaw. I should declare here and now that there were other reasons for my reluctance, not the least of which was the Scotch and champagne before takeoff. Despite my concerns, I could never deny my profession. Yet, I am more than happy to defer to some young buck eager to make an impression. My preferred role is always sage advisor and arch second-guesser. I have a healthy respect for the obstacle that teamwork presents to a couple of unacquainted physicians.

You guessed it. Nobody responded. There was another sandbagger on the flight. We met as we passed through the galley. After the usual preliminary questions about specialty he quickly begged off. He was retired, he said, and would prefer not to get involved. His guilt was palpable. This provoked a fleeting thought on my part about malpractice coverage in international skies. But I was committed now and not to be deterred. After all, this was what it was all about. My mother had announced to me early on, just following her decision that I become a physician, "Make sure you choose a specialty so that you can stand up at the country club when they call for a doctor." I never have been sure to which specialty she was referring, but I blame her that I am not a dermatologist today.

The supervising stewardess informed me that one of her flight attendants was "unresponsive." This sounded like a medical emergency to me. I was surprised at how calmly she proclaimed this. I attributed it to the kind of grace under pressure that one expects from the folks in the wild blue yonder. Trying to emulate her demeanor, I followed her to a perfectly normal-appearing uniformed attendant whom I recognized as the first person to serve me when I boarded the flight. She now appeared about the same, except that she seemed unwilling to speak. She had, I was told, gradually reached this condition over the period of an hour. She had become forgetful and slow and would do nothing but lean against the center divider with her arms folded across her chest. She appeared alert, had no gross evidence of a neurologic deficit, and was certainly in no distress. Still, there she was. I had to do something.

The Captain suggested that she might have suffered a stroke. The thought had not occurred to me. I quickly assured everyone that I had already eliminated that diagnosis. She was too young . . . too attractive. I prayed they would see logic where I could not. Nor did I know anything about this woman. It seems flight crews are not necessarily permanent teams but are often thrown together at the last moment; her colleagues could not help with any history. So here I stood, all eyes on me, and all ears hanging on every brilliant utterance (I was reminded of the old E.F. Hutton ad). I felt enormous pressure to say something profound. I asked her name. "Helga," I was told. After a few insipid questions to which I received nothing but Helga's icy stare, I decided I needed some time away from my audience to pull my thoughts together. I pronounced to the Captain that this was as close to veterinary medicine as I had been since forced to care for screaming children during a stint in the military. Helga had a look about her that reminded me of panic. Hers or my own, I cannot say. I informed the Captain that this appeared to be a stable situation and a more thorough examination risked the exposure of this potential panic I feared. "Then," I warned the Captain, "we'll have to tie her to the seat for 7 hours." The Captain quickly agreed; Helga was led quietly to her seat and strapped in. I mumbled something about the possibility of drugs or a psychological disorder and uneasily returned to my cold dinner.

Although I was assured by my retired colleague that my judgment was sound, I struggled with the problem and could think of nothing else for the next hour or so. I spotted one of the most helpful of the female attendants coming my way. It occurred to me to ask her if we could go through Helga's luggage. She was ahead of me. She came, she said, to show me Helga's purse. Imagine my little heart when we discovered the bottles and bottles of injectable insulin. I paused to allow my professional life to pass quickly before my eyes and commanded the attendant to direct me to my patient.

There was my Helga, the same bright stare, the cute smirk, but now in all its glory, the early stages of decerebrate rigidity. Just so that you have a clear vision of the situation, I should point out that I had a choice as I ministered to my patient. I could have sat next to her like a companion or I could be her physician and place myself in front of her. I bravely chose the latter. In order to accomplish that, I found myself kneeling on the floor in front of her. It was from this position that I made a pitiful effort to feed her orange juice, managing only to soak her blouse with the life-saving liquid. It was during the next few minutes as I was trying to work out the mechanics for an emergency orange juice enema that my stewardess/nurse/angel asked whether I was interested in reviewing the standard emergency medical kit. "I was just about to ask for such a kit," I said archly, and asked that she fetch it immediately. I felt my stewardess/nurse's confidence in me grow as I proceeded two steps behind her.

The emergency kit had an inventory printed on the case. The available light in our cubby did not allow my presbyopic eyes to read the print, but again my able assistant served me well. I could comment on the comprehensiveness of the kit, but our time would be better spent describing my mixture of feelings when the angel of the air uttered the precious words "50% dextrose and water." On the one hand, I was pleased that the cure for my patient was available. On the other hand, I must admit that my pleasure quickly turned to semi-panic as my thoughts raced to the certain confrontation I would soon have to face with that old devil, the venipuncture.

I must say I was once considered quite adept with the manual procedures one learns as a trainee, and later in my career was the procedurist of choice for those few procedures necessary to a nephrologist. Venipuncture is one thing, venipuncture on one's hands and knees, in a moving aircraft, done by a slightly rusty physician is quite another. My final delight came when I reviewed the package and found a 50-cc syringe with the needle connection dead in the center of the barrel. Now, in addition to my other concerns, I would have to forego the luxury of steadying the barrel on the limb, and would have to attack at about 35 degrees and at a moving target. I wanted to be someplace else.

The sweet, sterile liquid was drawn up, the tourniquet in place on the rigid left arm, a small vein palpable and visible just lateral to the antecubital fossa. At exactly this critical moment the pilot made the familiar announcement: "Ladies and gentlemen, we will experience a bit of turbulence for a few minutes." All of this in the usual reassuring drawl with which frequent fliers are so familiar. I hope the picture is clear.

Who is it that said, "I'd rather be lucky than good"? The needle found its way in very nicely. I aspirated a puff of the most gorgeous red blood I have ever seen and experienced euphoria. Now I carefully injected the glucose solution. No swelling appeared around the puncture site! At about the 35-cc mark I looked at Helga. How was she feeling, I asked. "I'm fine," she responded. The response of the hypoglycemic patient to intravenous glucose remains one of the most dramatic events in medicine. She was, in a matter of moments, virtually recovered.

It is a peripheral issue certainly, but of interest, that she denied taking any insulin, denied being a diabetic, and, in fact, was quite indignant when asked why she had insulin in her handbag. She insisted on returning to her station and even rejected German medical attention when they boarded the plane in Berlin. At my suggestion, the Captain arranged for her to be removed from the flight and to be observed by a physician in Berlin until she was out of danger.

I must say I enjoyed hero status for the balance of the flight and the acclaim has still not totally subsided, even today. During the check-in for my return flight I was flagged, placed in the VIP lounge, and humbly asked if I would accept first-class accommodations. In Berlin, the regional vice-president of the airline boarded the plane and presented me with an expensive bottle of Moët & Chandon, at the same time informing me that I would be hearing soon from corporate headquarters. Those who know me well will have no difficulty envisioning how graciously I accepted the praise and recognition. You and I know I didn't deserve it, but I have had some tribulations in the past few years and I didn't deserve them either. And I was beginning to learn how surgeons must feel and why their services are reimbursed as they are.

The irony is not subtle. Had this patient been brought to any emergency ward in the United States, she would have been given some intravenous glucose with no downside risk. Certainly the noble ER physician would not have received any recognition, unless of course he or she had not performed the simple but mandatory drill. The cognitive trick here is the review of the conditions that could be the cause of bizarre behavior, with special attention to those that are treatable. But I was being praised for successfully performing a simple procedure that was almost too late because I had missed the diagnosis. I blew the hard part and no one noticed.

My clearest thought in the aftermath was that this whole episode was a fascinating microcosm of the physician reimbursement debate. The airline personnel had emphatically come down on the side of the procedure. They were not the least bit concerned about my diagnostic prowess . . . or lack thereof. Rather, they were thrilled that I had successfully performed a procedure so simple that several people on the flight might have done it as well.

We are fascinated with the procedure. Praise to the person who can invade! Why no enthusiasm for making a diagnosis? I have a theory. Compare the size of the audience for public television's William F. Buckley program with that for televised sporting events. How about a heavyweight championship prizefight? The Super Bowl? The Indianapolis 500? We are an action-oriented society. Forget about thinking. The children of Plato now want blood. And they are willing to pay for it.

Then There Were None

THOMAS C. CONIGLIONE, MD
J. ARDEN BLOUGH, MD

On 19 April 1995 at 9:02 A.M., a terrorist bomb destroyed the Alfred P. Murrah Federal Office Building in Oklahoma City, Oklahoma. Within minutes, the disaster plan was activated at St. Anthony Hospital, the closest medical facility. At 9:08 A.M., the first victims arrived at the emergency room in pickup trucks, cars, and vans. A red Corvette with a blown-out windshield made several trips from the blast site to the emergency room, each time leaving a bleeding victim, then speeding off to pick up another. These initial victims were treated in the emergency room for various superficial injuries caused by flying glass.

By 9:18 A.M., the first ambulances arrived, transporting victims who had sustained major traumatic injuries. To make room for these victims, we moved the patients with superficial lacerations from the emergency room to an adjacent outpatient clinic area. Within the next 10 minutes, ambulances were arriving with such great frequency that three triage teams were required. Overflow of critically injured patients from the emergency room was sent to a nearby intensive care unit. Those less seriously injured were sent to the clinic area.

Ambulances arrived in groups of three or four, some carrying single victims with severe multiple injuries, others containing two to four less severely injured victims. All victims had lacerations from flying glass. The ambulance floors were sticky from the blood. Because the blast occurred at a time when many of the active staff physicians were in or near the hospital, most of the large number of physicians in the emergency room were from St. Anthony or the adjacent Bone and Joint Hospital.

With his entire head and eyes covered with bloody bandages, a young man wearing only a blood-stained T-shirt and Marine Corps uniform pants was helped out of the back door of an ambulance. Hospital staff carefully supported his each step. As he was helped into a wheelchair, one of the staff members leaned over and whispered in his ear, "You're going to be OK now, son." As the Marine was wheeled into the emergency room, the triaging physician summoned waiting ophthalmologists and general surgeons to his aid. We later learned this Marine, father of two and soon to be three, would no longer be able to serve in the Marine Corps as a jet pilot because of a traumatic injury to his right eye. The young Marine had been on the eighth floor of the federal building visiting Marine friends, as he did each month. After the blast, the friends to whom he had been speaking were nowhere to be found. Their bodies were later recovered. His poise and composure were so remarkable, we developed a new appreciation for the Marine Corps slogan "A Few Good Men."

A woman arrived whose hand was on a doorknob at the time of the blast. Compound fractures of the ulna and radius had been wrapped at the blast site. She was wheeled into the emergency room to a waiting orthopedist. A young man whose back was turned against a pane of glass in the federal building at the time of the blast was brought into the emergency room. Four hours later, through the efforts of three surgeons, the nearly 200 lacerations of his back, shoulders, and head had been cleansed and sutured. Two days later, more glass fragments were removed from his body.

Half a block away, a woman was on the fifth floor of a building across from the federal building. She was facing a window at the time of the explosion. A shard of glass pierced her neck. She was brought off the ambulance with a paramedic applying direct pressure to the right side of her neck. Nonetheless, blood was pouring out of her neck wounds. Hemoptysis indicated that her airway was compromised. Waiting cardiovascular and general surgeons rushed her to the operating room. Forty minutes later, they had repaired her transsected esophagus and the injuries to her carotid artery and jugular vein.

Telephone lines to the emergency room and treatment areas were jammed. Handheld radios provided extra communication among the physicians directing each treatment area. Radio communication enabled us to continually allocate physicians, nurses, supplies, and equipment to various areas. More importantly, we could remain aware of the capacity of each area to accept additional patients.

Somehow, with the sense of urgency as great as it was, steps and movement were efficient, voices and emotions were under control. Professionalism and decorum were evident everywhere. Even though the three triage teams were evaluating patients who were arriving more rapidly than one per minute, patient distribution and treatment were organized.

Between 9:30 and 9:45 A.M., the clinic areas began to overflow with patients. One nurse recognized the need to open an additional treatment area to accept the overflow. She selected a medical–surgical floor. With the assistance of hospital support staff, the entire floor was soon available as a treatment area, complete with suture sets, dressings, appropriate lighting, physicians, and nurses. Another spontaneous decision was to place patients with ocular injuries and ophthalmologists into another area. Throughout the day, hospital staff made many similar decisions that deviated from the established and well-rehearsed disaster plan, a plan that had seemed so rational before the event. However, the decisions made after the actual disaster were instinctive responses based on the circumstances, the needs of the moment, and an awareness of the hospital's resources. In retrospect, it was these decisions, made more collectively than through a defined chain of command, that enabled the hospital to respond to the enormous challenge of this disaster.

Contingency plans were formulated to use other areas of the hospital and to use the Bone and Joint Hospital if other treatment areas would be needed. Another area being prepared was the family medicine residency clinic, located in a professional office building adjacent to the hospital. However, a bomb threat closed that building for the rest of the day.

Because nonemergency surgeries had been canceled at 9:15 A.M., the operating rooms were available and well prepared. Between 9:45 and 10:00 A.M., three victims were already in operating rooms, each with a team of surgeons. The surgical suite was instructed to keep "two ORs ahead." Transportation of the injured to the operating rooms required that the gurneys pass through hallways that were becoming crowded with medical personnel. Volunteers, blood donors, and family members from across the city, the county, and even other parts of Oklahoma were streaming into every hospital entrance.

Conference rooms designated for family members rapidly became overcrowded. Family members, clergy, social workers, and psychiatrists were relocated to a large conference center in the hospital's mental health center. Food service employees served as a human chain of guides for visitors unfamiliar with the hospital.

To maintain organization in the emergency room, identification tags were used to designate the volunteers as "RN" or "MD." Each group was assigned to wait in a specific area anticipating the arrival of more injured persons. In the street in front of the emergency room entrance was stationed an employee holding a long pole high in the air. Mounted on the pole was a large arrow inscribed with "injured" pointing toward the emergency room entrance.

Because enough staff were available for treating patients at the hospital, triage teams were dispatched to the blast site, complete with physicians, nurses, and supplies. They rode in ambulances returning to the federal building. Before sitting in the patient compartments, they had to wipe the blood from the benches and walls.

Two nurses from one of the teams rescued a grandmother from a middle floor of the destroyed federal building. They wheeled her carrier out of an ambulance. It was reassuring to see them return safely.

The woman's fractured hip was surgically repaired. A young woman arrived in an ambulance with endotracheal tube in place, pupils dilated and fixed. The immediate computed tomographic scan showed multiple skull fractures, intraventricular hemorrhage, and marked cerebral edema. When her body was subsequently taken from the hospital to the medical examiner's office, we did not even know her name. During the day, five other Jane Does and one John Doe were treated and eventually identified.

All victims had glass embedded in their bodies, hair, and clothing. It was difficult to walk anywhere in the treatment areas without crunching glass underfoot. Once treatment was completed, victims searched for their families and asked about the status of other injured coworkers.

At 10:30 A.M., radio communication with the emergency medical service was lost, and television reports became the source of information. A police officer dispatched to the emergency medical service office located one block from the hospital complex learned that the service's broadcast frequency had been changed. Communication was eventually restored. Short-wave radio operators who were parked on the street outside the emergency room aided our security department in maintaining communication.

By now, six hospital areas, including the operating rooms, were being used for treatment. Each treatment area contained a portable radiograph unit. Pneumatic tubes provided laboratory results to the emergency room. Telephone lines remained overloaded. Radios and runners were still being used for internal communication. All nonemergency laboratory testing was postponed during the crisis, and qualified laboratory personnel were reassigned to blood-banking functions.

At 10:40 A.M., we were informed that a second bomb had been found at the federal building and that all rescuers had been instructed to evacuate the blast site. We were told to expect a second wave of as many as 200 casualties after deactivation of the bomb. While we anxiously waited, the hospital's food service staff began providing the first of 1700 sack lunches to the volunteers and family members. Local restaurants also pitched in with pizzas, sandwiches, and hamburgers for the waiting volunteers.

At approximately 11:30 A.M., in response to requests for updated information from the media and in an effort to stem the overwhelming flow of volunteers and blood donors, a news conference was held in front of the hospital.

By 1:00 P.M., the second bomb threat was determined to be a hoax. No second wave had materialized. Only a few injured survivors still trickled in, then there were none. Our anticipation yielded to frustration and helplessness as calls were received for body bags. Additional security officers were strategically placed at all entrances to prevent media access to the injured or to the families. As the disaster response was downgraded, most hospital personnel returned to their regular duties. Residents from the St. Anthony Hospital family practice residency program who were no longer actively involved in treatment were dispatched throughout the hospital to systematically reevaluate and coordinate the care of the injured persons admitted to the hospital. In the emergency room, however, extra staff maintained a heightened state of readiness throughout the afternoon and evening. Some treatment areas were busy late into the night.

More than 400 family members had crowded into the conference room designated as the family center. Throughout the day, families were provided information as our hospital staff communicated with other hospitals through fax machines. Taped to the walls of the family members' conference room were large poster-sized lists containing handwritten names of injured persons being treated at St. Anthony and other area hospitals. Hospital staff constantly updated the lists. As the afternoon wore on, family members who could not find their loved ones' names on the lists grew more anxious and despondent.

A bank of telephones was installed for use by family members. After the local media broadcast these numbers, the telephones never ceased ringing with inquiries from across Oklahoma, the United States, and the world. St. Anthony staff researched each of these hundreds of inquiries and returned each telephone call, working late into the night.

With darkness descending on the bomb site, hundreds of visitors anxiously searched for their missing loved ones, circulating among hospital emergency rooms with pictures clutched in their hands. One family wanted to search the entire hospital, room by room, to find a missing family member.

Simultaneously, media from across the country descended on Oklahoma City. Most were overwhelmed by the enormity of the human carnage; some were looking for an exposé. Hospital officials were especially careful to ensure the privacy of the victims and their families.

Late in the evening, instructions were received from the state medical examiner's office that all remaining family members were to proceed to a local church, which had become the official information site for families. By this time, many of the families had established a bond with the hospital staff or with some of the volunteer staff. We reluctantly complied with the instructions and announced that families were to proceed to the church. Even more reluctantly, they departed.

During the first day, eight patients were treated in the operating rooms. Multiple procedures were done by 36 surgeons. At one point, five patients were having surgical procedures simultaneously. During the first day, six ruptured globes were repaired, 50 units of blood were transfused, and the hospital's entire supply of plasma expanders (hetastarch) was used.

One patient whom we later learned was almost declared dead at the scene had 9.5 hours of surgery, performed by 11 surgeons. Her husband had been to each area hospital with her photograph several times. No one could identify his wife as a victim being treated. On his fourth visit to St. Anthony, a hospital nurse could not identify her photo as one of our Jane Does. However, she noticed that the man's wedding band was identical to that of a Jane Doe. Two days later, the patient had another 7.5 hours of plastic surgery. Five days later, she awakened from a coma. Three weeks later, appearing miraculously improved but still disfigured, she was discharged from the hospital.

Within 24 hours of the disaster, crisis intervention teams were mobilized to provide assistance to hospital staff who were deemed to be at the highest risk for psychological trauma from the disaster.

*　　*　　*　　*

In subsequent days, individual counseling was provided to all hospitalized victims and to most of those treated and released, as well as their families. More than 600 hospital employees underwent debriefing.

In subsequent days, physicians counseled each other. Each of us felt an uncomfortable gnawing sense of not having done enough.

In subsequent days, we treated injured firefighters and rescue workers from around the country. They often delayed their treatment because of their reluctance to interrupt their teams' rescue efforts. By interacting with them, we developed a new appreciation for the words "dedication" and "bravery."

In subsequent days, our tears reflected both compassionate sorrow and admiration for the bravery and generosity of the community and the country.

In subsequent days, we learned that caring and kindness were stronger than hatred and destruction.

At Ease

RONALD H. LANDS, MD

The suit he wore, purchased years before, fluttered on his angular frame like a flag on July 4th. The dark hollows around his eyes were a haunting contrast to the shock of thick white hair that he combed straight back from his forehead. The manicured nails did not disguise that several of his fingers had been broken and allowed to heal without intervention. A polished hickory walking cane hung like an ornament over his crooked left arm as he limped back and forth across the length of my examining room.

I was late, but he camouflaged his impatience. Every question I asked him, he answered with the soldierly addition of "Sir" to the end of each sentence. I extracted the history of his present illness painfully. I would ask a question, only to hear him rephrase it and minimize the answer.

"Yes, Sir. I may have lost some weight, Sir."

"How much do you think you may have lost?"

"Over how long, Sir?"

"How much have you lost over the last 2 months?"

"Oh, I'm not sure. Probably 30 or 40 pounds, but I needed to lose some of it, Sir. I was getting a bit heavy."

His past medical history was even more global and even more

brief. "I was involved in some trauma back in '66," he explained when I asked about the obvious disability he had acquired from his many broken bones.

A little frustrated, I moved to the physical exam. A screaming eagle glared at me from its tattooed perch on his right shoulder while I examined his axillae for adenopathy. I recognized it as the unit crest of a U.S. Army infantry division, and I wondered when he had served. The esprit implied in that eagle stood out in sharp relief on his deformed and cachectic arm.

I scheduled several scans for the following morning. I walked through the radiology department that same morning, timing my visit to when I hoped the results would be available. Instead, I found my patient, standing as rigidly at attention as his deformed limbs would allow, at the hub of a helpless circle of radiology personnel. He had fixed his eyes on a focal point far away.

"Sir. I will not get back into that box," he said as I walked into the room.

"He's claustrophobic," I explained pedantically to the group. "The confining dimensions of the scanner must frighten him." With humiliating doses of sedatives, I made him sleep through the scans.

Back in my office the following day, he had no memory of the scanner incident. He listened intently while I explained the diagnostic implications of anemia, adenopathy, fevers, sweats, and weight loss. He acknowledged my treatment recommendations as if they were operations orders for some military mission. His eyes, once again, disengaged briefly.

"Let's get started," he said.

Over the next few months, an uninterrupted spiral of therapy, followed by toxicity, followed by tumor recurrence whittled relentlessly at his pride. During the last of several hospital admissions, he developed an agitated delirium. Mistaking his intravenous tubing for shackles, he exhausted himself with efforts to "escape and evade." He tried to defend himself from a nurse who startled him while administering his medicine. The delirium cleared slowly and without explanation. Emotionally exhausted after that experience, he decided to forego any further chemotherapy. I did not argue with him.

During one of his last visits to my office, he brought two documents for me to read. The first was an article published in a small-town newspaper in June 1968. The yellowed pages announced, **LOCAL HERO RETURNS AFTER FOURTEEN MONTHS IN A PRISONER OF WAR CAMP.** A fellow prisoner had described for the reporter an occasion during which their captors punished my hero by isolating him in a small wooden box. With his knees to his chest, and his arms wrapped around his broken legs, he survived, inexplicably, for days. When finally released, he vowed to his comrades that he would die before enduring "the box" again.

The second manuscript was a notarized copy of his living will. It outlined the usual legalistic points concerning tube feeding, mechanical ventilation, and cardiac resuscitation. He had additionally directed, in meticulous print, that his body be cremated and the ashes scattered from the arches of an ancient bridge spanning a tributary of the Tennessee River.

He watched me, intently, until I finished reading. His eyes locked on mine as he folded the papers and put them in his briefcase.

"Don't let them put me in a box, Sir," he said.

In a flash of understanding, the many times I had unwittingly caused him to relive the horrors of that prison camp passed vividly through my mind.

"At ease, Soldier," I said. "It's the least I can do."

WANTED: 21st Century Physician

FAITH T. FITZGERALD, MD

Altruistic, compassionate, courageous, intellectually curious, frugal scholar, gifted in history, philosophy, politics, economics, sociology, and psychology. Must have working knowledge of biology, chemistry, physics, and medicine. Physical endurance, emotional maturity, and technical-manual skills sufficient to take apart and reassemble the human body and mind at levels ranging from the micromolecular to the gross are required; must have flexibility to master all knowledge, sift and discard that no longer applicable, while discovering new data at the bench, in clinical practice, in both general and subspecialty medicine. Teaching, counseling, administrative, computer, and budgetary expertise essential, as is commitment to the disenfranchised. A working knowledge of the law; literary, artistic, and musical talent; and multilingualism highly desirable. Should be able to prevent and cure disease, including the depredations of advancing age; physical disarray; and spiritual, mental, emotional, and economic illnesses. Will need to function effectively and efficiently in both intensive care units and urban slums.

Salary ideally should be no issue, though heavy initial investment by the candidate is required. Benefits variable, depending on the individual's principal source of gratification. This is a 24 hour per day commitment.

Should make house calls.

It Should Once Again See Light

BLAIR P. GRUBB, MD

Several years ago, a physician from southern France contacted me. His granddaughter had taken ill with a disease that baffled the physicians there. He called after reading several of my articles on disorders of the autonomic nervous system. His granddaughter's symptoms seemed to match those I had described, and he asked me if I could help. I readily agreed, and for many months, I collaborated with the child's French physicians by telephone and by fax, directing their diagnostic testing. At last we came to a diagnosis, and I prescribed a course of therapy. During the next several weeks, the child made a seemingly miraculous recovery. Her grandparents expressed their heartfelt thanks and told me to let them know should I ever come to France.

In the summer of 1996, I was invited to speak at a large international scientific meeting that was to be held in Nice, France. I sent word to the physician I had helped years before. Upon my arrival at the hotel, I received a message to contact him. I called him, and we arranged a night to meet for dinner.

On the appointed day we met and then drove north to his home in the beautiful southern French countryside. It was humbling to learn his home was older than the United States. During the drive he told me that his wife had metastatic breast cancer and was not well, but she insisted upon meeting me. When introduced to her, I saw that despite her severe illness, she was still a beautiful woman with a noble bearing.

I was thereafter treated to one of the most wonderful meals I have ever eaten, complemented by the most exquisite of wines. After dinner, we sat in a 17th-century salon, sipping cognac and chatting. Our conversation must have seemed odd to the young man and woman who served us because it came out in a free-flowing mixture of English, French, and Spanish. After a time the woman asked, "My husband tells me you are Jewish, no?" "Yes," I said, "I am a Jew." They asked me to tell them about Judaism, especially the holidays. I did my best to explain and was astounded by how little they knew of Judaism. She seemed to be particularly interested in Hanukkah. Once I had finished answering her questions, she suddenly looked me in the eye and said, "I have something I want to give to you." She disappeared and returned several moments later with a package wrapped in cloth. She sat, her tired eyes looking into mine, and she began to speak slowly.

"When I was a little girl of 8 years, during the Second World War, the authorities came to our village to round up all the Jews. My best friend at that time was a girl of my age named Jeanette. One morning when I came to play, I saw her family being forced at gunpoint into a truck. I ran home and told my mother what had happened and asked where Jeanette was going. 'Don't worry,' she said, 'Jeanette will be back soon.' I ran back to Jeanette's house only to find that she was gone and that the other villagers were looting her home of valuables, except for the Judaic items, which were thrown into the street. As I approached, I saw an item from her house lying in the dirt. I picked it up and recognized it as an object that Jeanette and her family would light around Christmas time. In my little girl's mind I said 'I will take this home and keep it for Jeanette, till she comes back,' but she and her family never returned."

She paused and took a slow sip of brandy. "Since that time I have kept it. I hid it from my parents and didn't tell a soul of its existence.

Indeed, over the last 50 years the only person who knew of it was my husband. When I found out what really happened to the Jews, and how many of the people I knew had collaborated with the Nazis, I could not bear to look at it. Yet I kept it, hidden, waiting for something, although I wasn't sure what. Now I know what I was waiting for. It was you, a Jew, who helped cure our granddaughter, and it is to you I entrust this."

Her trembling hands set the package on my lap. I slowly unwrapped the cloth from around it. Inside was a menorah, but one unlike any I had seen before. Made of solid brass, it had eight cups for holding oil and wicks and a ninth cup centered above the others. It had a ring attached to the top, and the woman mentioned that she remembered that Jeanette's family would hang it in the hallway of their home. It looked quite old to me; later, several people told me that it is probably at least 100 years old. As I held it and thought about what it represented, I began to cry. All I could manage to say was a garbled "merci." As I left, her last words to me were "Il faudra voir la lumière encore une fois"—it should once again see light.

I later learned that she died less than 1 month after our meeting. This Hanukkah, the menorah will once again see light. And as I and my family light it, we will say a special prayer in honor of those whose memories it represents. We will not let its lights go out again.

There But for Fortune

KAREN E. VICTOR, MD

At the end of the first day of the Society of General Internal Medicine meeting in San Diego, I got into a taxi to go to my hotel. The driver was a thin, tired-looking, middle-aged man who spoke in gentle, accented English.

After some talk about the weather and where I was from, I asked him how long he'd been in the States.

"A year and a half," he said.

"Welcome."

"Thanks, ma'am."

He had come from Afghanistan.

He asked if I was a physician, and then what the conference was about.

Well, I said, it was about how to be a better physician and a better teacher of physicians-in-training. We were trying to learn how to use questions and physical examination more thoughtfully and how to do fewer unnecessary tests.

"You mean not getting an MRI on the first day?"

"Exactly."

We talked a little more. When he used the word "symptomatology," I asked him what his work had been in Afghanistan.

He had been a surgeon.

"You know, ma'am, I have no health insurance here. One day my son had a pharyngitis, and I took him to the emergency room. We waited a long time, of course, and then a physician saw him. I think he was a resident. He did a test and then said my son had β-hemolytic streptococcal infection. He prescribed cephalexin. It is a broad-spectrum antibiotic, yes? I asked him, 'Excuse me, why do you not use penicillin?' The physician got very angry, tore up the prescription, and yelled at me, 'If you're a doctor, you can prescribe him the penicillin! If not, you need to shut up and let me be the doctor!'"

"I agree with you completely about the penicillin," I said, "but even if you were wrong, nobody should be treated that rudely."

"Ma'am," my taxi driver continued, "In my country, during the war, I had to do eight amputations, below-the-knee, in one night. These are very difficult, you know. And I never, ever lost my temper like that."

He missed being a physician, and hoped someday to be licensed here. For the time being, he drove a taxi so that he and his family could eat.

He was grateful to be in a country that is not at war.

The Prison Patient

MATTHEW D.S. KLEIN, MD

Bennett drove to the state prison in the last moments before dawn. A second-year resident went to the prison at this promising hour every day of the year, and Bennett liked the drive. Long before other cars lit up the freeway with a dazzling headlight show, Bennett rolled his pickup truck down the entrance ramp and onto the empty night road. He kept his window down to touch and breathe the air. When he switched lanes, his turn signal blinked through the blue night like a satellite, and Bennett rocketed toward the great floodlit towers of the prison, glowing in the empty country.

Inside the prison, the lights were repellent, and the same air felt chilly and damp. Cheryl, the nurse, brought him a cup of coffee. Bennett fell into his chair in the little concrete office. He leaned back, legs spread wide like a high-school football coach, and flipped the list over. Only one name was on the roster.

"Only one today, hey," he said, still flipping at the corner of the list.

"Oh yes. Did you see who it is?" said Cheryl.

"Masterson? Oh boy." Bennett knew Masterson from other days. He came often. "Well, bring him in," he said, although the deputy had gone to retrieve the prisoner when he heard Bennett's heels coming down the hall.

"This is Masterson's last visit," Cheryl said. "He's going to court today. He's getting out." She was sure about this. In fact, Bennett trusted her to know more about these things than the law partners or the reporters because her mundane daily workload depended on the outcome. He was rarely surprised. Cheryl knew which prisoners went home from court.

There was a slam of the steel bolts in the doors. The deputy's voice rang through the office. "Stand along the left wall, Masterson. Atta boy. Siddown." The deputy appeared in the door, looking down at his slip of paper. He held it low on his abdomen and squinted at it over a spectacular jaw and chest. "I got your man," he said, and as he looked up, his flat top moved to a perfect horizontal. Cheryl nodded, and the deputy ducked into the next room for a cup of coffee.

"Mr. Masterson, come on in," Bennett said, waving his arm. He pressed his right hand into the chair between his legs and brought himself into a sitting position. Masterson, 62 years old, had suffered a heart attack about 6 months earlier. He came to see Bennett at the prison clinic almost every other day with an urgent concern. At first, Bennett had been spooked by Masterson, but the inmate was gentle with him, and respectful, and these qualities in someone so rough and different from himself stirred a kind of caring in Bennett's heart.

And Masterson needed Dr. Bennett. The heart attack 6 months ago haunted him incessantly as he plodded through the hours of windowless rooms and television, of foul language and urine, of farts and fights and humiliation.

He had been a car repairman before prison. Sometimes it seemed that he came to Bennett just to talk about cars, to get his mind off of his heart. No one had ever talked to Bennett about cars. He would describe a Monte Carlo engine, round and humming and shining, and compare it to a lady's smooth leg just where it flares into a buttock. He would shoot Bennett a sideways grin, then look down, ashamed. When Bennett glanced reflexively at the clock, Masterson would catch it and get to the point. He would ask Bennett about a mole on his belly, or a bump on his elbow, or a twinge that he had felt in his shoulder while watching "Baywatch." The inmate had a thousand nonexistent lesions, all imagined tangents from his heart. Bennett would listen to his lungs and listen to his belly, squeeze his lumpy shoulders and pat him on the back. When he reassured Masterson, when he said pointedly, "Your heart sounds fine, Mr. Masterson," the inmate would cry, big and jerky and trying to stop. After the deputy took him back to his cell, Bennett often sat quietly, impressed by his own unexpected power and by the transparency of Masterson's soul.

One day after the patient had left, Bennett overheard the deputy mutter, "Yeah, stay good and healthy so you can go bugger some more little boys, Masterson." The grin on Bennett's face suddenly fell. His sympathy for the criminal seemed repulsive. Later, he stole a chance to review his patient's computer file and, when no one was looking, flipped the screen to the criminal record. Fifth-degree sexual assault. Sex with a minor. Distribution of child pornography. Sex with a 12-year-old boy. Statutory rape. The screen rolled over for a few seconds, blinking with the size of the list. Each name was a victim, each number was a sweaty boy lying in bed, still waking in a nocturnal panic. Bennett's mouth went dry when he recalled the reassuring touches he had given Masterson; on his back, his legs, his face.

Masterson appeared in the door. He wore neat prison scrubs stretched over his broad belly and, as always, he wore his brown work boots with years of engine oil smeared across their tongues. "Good morning, Dr. Bennett," he said. He scratched at a piece of fuzz caught in his graying beard. "Dr. Bennett, can I talk to you alone today?" he said, and threw a couple of abashed looks at Cheryl.

"Yeah, certainly, Mr. Masterson," Bennett said, and as he motioned for Cheryl to leave he rolled his eyes just a little for her, and she giggled. But he felt his mouth go dry again, and felt his pulse beating in his throat. "What's going on?"

"Dr. Bennett," the inmate said, "that medicine you gave me keeps me from getting hard-ons." His voice broke. "I haven't even got it up in the morning for 2 months. Is there something wrong with me? I can't get it up, Dr. Bennett, and it's been ever since I started that pill."

Bennett had started Masterson on a β-blocker after the heart attack. He had forgotten to mention the possibility of impotence as a side effect. Back then, his patient's sex life hadn't occurred to him. "I don't want to take that pill any more, Dr. Bennett," he said, and his husky shoulders shook with real fear. "Am I sick? Am I going to die?" Masterson peeked up at him, shyly pulling up his shirt so Bennett could listen to his heart.

There was not even a pause. "Mr. Masterson, that pill is *saving* your life. You hear me? Listen to me." Bennett stood up and pulled his face close to the bearded, teary man. "Do you want another heart attack? Is that what you want? That pill is the only thing between you and the big one, see? Masterson, do you want to live to see tomorrow?" He was hissing at his patient and couldn't stop despite the petrified look in the man's eyes. Masterson nodded a tiny nod. "That pill is the only reason you are still alive today! That's the way it is, Masterson. You stick with that pill, every day. Hard-ons or no hard-ons," Bennett said, struggling not to sneer, "you take that pill."

There was a long silence, and Bennett heard only his own heart surging in his ears. "Can you listen to my heart today, Dr. Bennett?" the patient whispered. For the first time, Bennett thought he smelled something forbidden on Masterson's breath. His nostrils recoiled.

"Your heart is fine." Bennett said quietly, turning away. "For now."

When Bennett stepped out onto the highway again, the light was lifting to a unifying gray. A crowd of headlights danced furiously past. He leaned a hairy hand on the bed of his pickup, hung his head, and waited for his knees to stop shaking. Up in the sky, the old towers of the prison revealed more cracks and dust with each onrushing minute of daylight.

From an Observer

BONNIE B. SMITH, PHD

I teach virology to second-year medical students. In my job as an educator, I try to present information my students will need to function as competent doctors. But at times I wonder if I can determine what they need to know. I often ask myself if I include information truly important or only of interest to basic scientists like myself. When I teach Virology, for instance, I know that for my students to understand viral replication they must understand macromolecular synthesis. I am comfortable teaching that material. But how much of that do they need to know? What will they use in practice? Because I am not a physician, to some degree I am unable to answer.

Another aspect that troubles me about teaching medical students is lecturing on the clinical manifestations of viral diseases. That's where I am a fish out of water. For me, these diseases are merely descriptions in a book. They have no faces. It troubles me that I lecture on serious illnesses about which I have only read. How can I teach what I have never seen? My own children have not had chickenpox, and although I have, I did not observe the three types of lesions present simultaneously on my skin. Yet I teach it. I teach a lot about AIDS when I have no experiential knowledge of this disease.

For some time I had considered a way to remedy this deficiency. I wrote to an infectious disease specialist, requesting to join him on rounds for a few weeks. But then I set the letter aside. What was I afraid of? *Doctors* for one thing. I knew what they were really like. Physicians refer to patients by their diseases, not by their names. They are arrogant and abusive to residents on their service. What if they asked *me* questions? My second fear was just as irrational. I had seldom been around sick people. And the times that I have, I did not conduct myself very well. What if it happened again?

I spent a month mentally preparing myself. At last, I mailed the letter and went to the hospital, finally seeing patients with some of the diseases I had taught about for years. The suffering of patients afflicted with those maladies touched me deeply. This story is about just a few of the patients. It's also a story of my own growth and my glimpse on being a doctor.

On the first morning, I waited in the hospital lobby to meet Dr. Brewer, my stomach in knots. He arrived, we shook hands and I thought, "He seems pleasant; so far, so good." The first patients I saw were in the intensive care unit. We went first to a central work station where the charts were located. As Dr. Brewer reviewed a chart, I looked around at the darkened, glass-sided rooms with beds where people lay attached to tubes and IVs. There was a hum of machinery and a flickering of lights from TV sets families watched in patients' rooms while they waited for a miracle to happen.

Dr. Brewer explained about Mr. Hall, who had been in a car accident and had numerous injuries. He had been on the unit for several months and had had a fever for weeks. His condition was deteriorating. I looked over to the room as Dr. Brewer spoke. Mr. Hall appeared to be in his sixties. Although his eyes were open, he seemed unaware of his surroundings. A man stood over his bed, his son I presumed, speaking loudly, as though the volume of his words could penetrate his father's consciousness.

"You stay with us now," he said, his voice shaking, "You stay with us."

With a lump in my throat, I turned back to Dr. Brewer as he talked of the bacteria they had isolated and the antibiotics he was taking. I thought for the first of many times,

"My God, how do you do this?"

Leaving the intensive care unit, we walked up the stairs discussing Roberto, the next patient we were about to see. Dr. Brewer always told me their names and, often, a few details of their life. It was clear he knew them not just as patients but as people. I began to think that my image of physicians was not entirely correct.

Roberto was the first of many patients with AIDS that I saw. He was hospitalized with pneumocystis pneumonia. Allergic to trimethoprim-sulfamethoxazole, he was receiving intravenous pentamidine and was recovering from the pneumonia very slowly. I wrote all this down in my notebook. By focusing on the facts, I could escape the emotions I was trying not to feel. Roberto was propped up in bed, receiving oxygen. His chest heaved, his nostrils flared, and his sentences were punctuated by gasps every few words. As he talked, he looked from Dr. Brewer to me and back again. He must have thought I was another physician.

"Don't look horrified," I thought. "He thinks you're a doctor! Try to look compassionate . . . or is it empathetic?"

Our eyes met, I smiled, and thought, "Not that smile, that's the pity smile." Roberto knew it too and turned away.

It was then that I began to watch the way Dr. Brewer interacted with his patients. He had a calm demeanor, and it seemed as if he could look into their eyes and tell them something beyond the words he spoke. I thought that if I just watched him, I could try to give the same nonverbal message he did. It wasn't quite so easy, as I found when I met Adam.

Adam, Dr. Brewer explained, was "a nice young man, a solid citizen." He said that about quite a few people. Brewer told me Adam was a textbook example of what AIDS can do to a person. He had had diarrhea for the past few months and, thus, had lost 40 pounds. We talked about what might be the cause, which had not yet been determined. I knew this stuff! I had read many articles about this! I was thinking cryptosporidiosis or cytomegalovirus or maybe. . . . Then I saw him.

Adam Higgens was not much more than a skeleton. The skin was stretched tight over his gaunt face. His large brown eyes were sunk deep into their sockets. Still, his face showed that he had once been a handsome youth. I had a lump in my throat again. My thoughts raced back to 10 years ago. I was a graduate student. Paul Schnurin, one of the faculty members in our department, was hospitalized with a mysterious ailment affecting his entire gastrointestinal system. I visited him shortly after he went into the hospital, bringing some chocolate. That was my first mistake. Weeks become months, and he was still in the hospital. His family and I were members of the same church; I spoke to his wife on occasion. Like so many of us who meant well, I said I was sure he would get better. Everyone was praying. He had to get better. But the robust man I had known as teacher and scientist became horribly thin and frail, much the way Adam looked. Visiting Paul again, I stood at the entrance to his room, horrified. Tears came to my eyes, but they were not tears for him. They were a response to fear. Overcome with shock, I ran from the room. Now as I looked at Adam, those memories washed over me again. This time I could not run.

I had spent 2 weeks at the hospital when I saw Chris. He too had AIDS. Before this latest illness, he was an exceedingly intelligent and successful young man. Now he had neurologic symptoms from lymphoma in the brain and was receiving radiation treatments. The curtains in his room were closed, creating a somber appearance despite the bright summer day. The air was warm and heavy, and I noticed a faint odor of perspiration. Chris was curled on his side in his bed, his hair flattened against his head from sleep. His puffy face made him look childlike. In his arms he held a teddy bear.

Dr. Brewer stood by his bed. The radiation treatments did not seem to be working. "We'll try a few other things," he said, trying to sound hopeful.

Chris said nothing. He stared at the wall, holding the teddy bear tighter, as Dr. Brewer spoke.

I thought of my lecture on neurologic complications of AIDS. I teach about AIDS dementia complex, caused by the virus itself. Lymphomas I include almost as an afterthought. On a darkened stage in front of 160 students, I saw myself lecturing callously about diseases, detached from the people suffering from them. I could hear myself saying stolidly,

"Similar symptoms may be caused by primary lymphomas of the central nervous system . . . ."

That was all the time I spent on the subject. Yet here before me was a young man with "primary lymphoma of the central nervous system," one who should have so much more of his life left to live, and he was dying. Part of me wanted to stay with him, so he would not be alone. It occurred to me suddenly that I no longer felt overwhelmed by the urge to retreat from the suffering I saw. I was making progress.

I am back at my desk now, sheltered by books and journals as before. The goal of the weeks I spent on rounds was certainly met—I saw some of the maladies on which I lecture, and now I speak about these diseases with more confidence. But I am not the same. The experience has changed me. I had never before seen people clinging precariously to life. Pain and suffering were a reality whose existence I had tried to deny. Even a brief exposure to these patients' utter vulnerability caused me to lose some of my naiveté. I have a fresh admiration for the job of physicians and particularly for my students as I think of them caring for people in physical and emotional turmoil. It is an awesome responsibility.

Doctor's Daughter

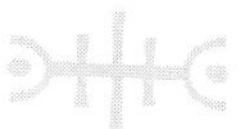

JULIA E. McMURRAY, MD

As a small child, I often stood on the stairway in my home, looking up at the pictures of my mother. O.U. School of Medicine, Class of 1945. I counted the 69 sepia-toned faces many times, always coming back to my mother's in the oval composite photograph. My mother is one of only three women, and her countenance is serious and composed; the hair in a long, wavy cut typical of the period. In an old picture from the local newspaper, written the year before my birth, my mother is sitting at a desk, wearing a white lab coat, staring out at the camera from her desk at the sexually transmitted diseases clinic where she worked. "Young Doctor Works in Town," reads the headline.

"How come you never worked as a doctor, Mama?" I asked frequently. I often went on rounds with my physician-father in the early morning at the community hospital in the small southern town where we lived. In one minute flat, he could tap a chest, letting the straw-colored liquid rush through the brown rubber tubing to puddle in the glass vacuum bottle on the bed. The nurses stood by at attention, in their starched white dresses and peaked caps. In the small emergency area, my father would casually flip his tie over his shoulder and insert the needle for the lumbar puncture that would diagnose the subarachnoid bleeding in his patient. Afterwards, we would drive home to the house, where my mother would be standing in front of the stove, scrambling eggs for my three brothers, who sat watching Saturday morning cartoons. My mother was always home.

"Well, I loved you children and felt you needed me at home." The answer was always the same. "You would start sucking your thumbs or the babysitter would quit." On the day I was born in an army barracks hospital, a psychotic WAC ran amok in the maternity area brandishing a butcher knife. My mother hid me behind her body next to the wall and called my father to come take us home. Later on, a German war-bride would sometimes babysit for my brother and me in a pinch so my mother could work. After the war, while my father was in fellowship training, there was a job for her at the public health department. The syphilis patients would sit on a long row of stools with their hospital gowns open in the back while she went from one to the other, performing the lumbar punctures for diagnosis or test of cure. It was the last clinical job she ever had.

Such were the stories of my childhood. In the small town near the mountains, my father worked first in solo practice, then with a gradually increasing number of partners. He was on call every second or third night for most of my childhood, and was rarely home. The special office phone at home, one that we were never to answer, ran off the hook each call night. Ventricular tachycardia, acute myocardial infarctions, diabetic ketoacidosis, and acute leukemia were never discussed at the dinner table but were nonetheless an integral part of the household. His cotton shirts were ironed every afternoon, and a sandwich was always waiting on the table for the 20-minute lunch break he took every day as he read his mail. On Sunday afternoons, I would go into the office with him while he saw patients. Using his secret name for me, I would pick up the phone and say gleefully, "Doctor McMurray's office, Miss Bird speaking," to neighbors and patients who knew me only as a quiet, well-behaved child.

My mother, on the other hand, was at home for us every day after school, cooking dinner in the evenings when my father walked in after rounds. She kept the family in clothes, helped with homework, played music to dance to on rainy afternoons, ferried us all to swimming and music lessons, met with the teacher when my brothers got into trouble at school, and always made it to recitals. She was president of the local mental health society, gave the embarrassing sex talks in schools, and thrilled us all once with a hole-in-one on the golf course. A gifted amateur naturalist, she admonished me not to be squeamish while helping me dissect fish eyes at the lake in the summers. Almost none of the other women in her circle of friends worked; most had never been to college. In the evenings she read all the "Great Books," and she loved nonfiction on almost any subject. I would crawl around her under the covers as she lay reading in bed, feeling the safety and security of her body.

The first crack in her armor of stoicism came when Betty Friedan's *The Feminine Mystique* was published. After reading the book, she refused to cook dinner for 3 days. She looked at me that afternoon and said, "I was smart; I could have done some things." I urged her to work out a way to drive the 3 hours to the nearest medical school in the state in order to get back into practice. But there were four children at home and one demanding, full-time private practice to support. Secretly, I chided my father for what I took to be his inflexibility in this regard; my mother simply said it couldn't be done.

I grew up, did well in school, and was a pre-medicine major in college. My father was emphatic in his support and unambivalent in his enthusiasm for medicine. "It's a great job. Easy, really. You just hang up your shingle and do things any way you like. People will come to see a woman physician. I wish your mother could have done it."

My mother was more cautious. "Whatever you want to do is fine; don't do it for me."

"How did you decide to become a doctor?" I once asked.

She responded in her typical low-key way, "I grew up in dust-bowl Oklahoma in the middle of the Depression. We had no money whatsoever. My father ran a garage, but I went to the state university. I was a chemistry major planning on going to pharmacy school, when a local couple urged me to go on to medical school. It was pretty simple, really. I just did it."

When my letter of acceptance came from medical school, she sent me a medical dictionary inscribed, "From one to another." Once in my clinical years, I began using her battered brown medical bag. Medical school was overwhelming, but memories of time spent with my father on house calls and in his office sustained me. I fell in and out of love a half dozen times, married during my residency, and ultimately started a family. My first job was exciting and utterly absorbing. Before the baby came, I was in every morning at 7:00 A.M., staying until late at night. No part-time work for me! Child care would be easy in the city where I lived, and my physician-husband was deeply committed to being involved as a father. It would all work out so easily. Why couldn't my mother have done this? I emulated my father at this point. My profession came first.

When my 4-month-old began reaching for his child care person instead of me and started sucking his thumb, I felt he needed me, as we had needed my mother. I cut back to part-time. Sitting with my child on my lap, I asked my mother, "Couldn't you have worked part-time?" This time, the stories were about the refusal of all the practices in town to hire anyone less than full-time. In fact, the only acceptable full-time jobs for women in her social strata were those of teacher or nurse. It wasn't considered acceptable otherwise.

My second child was born, and life got more complex. I would feel crazed with worry and guilt when a waiting room full of patients were waiting for me at the hospital while I sat helplessly in the pediatrician's office with a sick child. The nannies didn't want to work more than 8 to 10 hours a day, and the consultants always seemed to page me in the late afternoon while I was swinging the children out in the back yard. It was difficult to discuss the cardiac ejection fractions of patients receiving chemotherapy with the children squabbling in the background. As I contemplated my own difficulties, I seemed to be headed down the same road as my mother, and began to think more and more about the mystery of her lost medicine. I couldn't believe things had been so cut and dried, so matter of fact. How could she have avoided the gut-wrenching feelings of guilt, love, and inadequacy that I myself so often felt? And so I became instantly alert one hot summer day, as I sat by a pool with my mother and watched my two small children swim.

The question was innocent enough. "So, Mom, just how far did you get in residency exactly? What kind of doctor were you planning to be?"

At her answer I felt a sudden stillness, the sounds of the summer cicadas buzzing loudly in my ears. "I wanted to be a pediatrician, but I got sick."

Sick? My mother was robustly healthy and had not been sick a day in her life. "What do you mean sick, Mother? What kind of sick?"

She answered, "It was stress, I guess." And for the first time she told me the story of how she started in a pediatric residency during the war. Four men, one woman. All the men were married and lived with their families. My mother was given a small room for living quarters on the tuberculosis ward. Being skin-test negative, she was terrified of contracting tuberculosis and asked to be moved. She was then put in a room at the end of the hall in the nurses' quarters. "It was just too much," my mother said in a voice devoid of emotion. She moved to the town where her sister lived, met my father, and married. There it was. A shaky start in the profession: scared, unsupported, possibly unwanted in medicine. The other answer had been in front of me all my life: the demands of mothering, needs of a busy physician-husband, a reluctant profession, and small-town social mores that made employment difficult for a woman physician who wanted a home in addition to a career.

My father retired at the age of 62. After 40 years of working, he told me that he hadn't had a summer off since the third grade. A poem came from him once that said, "I wish I had picked more daisies." Although he would say that he had been more successful than he had ever dreamed, in other moments he would speak of "being sucked dry" by patients or mention feats and anxieties that kept him awake at night, shared with no one. My mother would bask in the glories of her grandchildren and never once mention her lost medicine.

As for me, I have come through. I am fortunate to have been able to work part-time and to have a physician-husband willing and able to be fully engaged as a partner in our enterprise of work and home. But the challenges have been formidable, and not simply a matter of more child care, more housecleaning help, or take-out food. Childrens' needs are not always so easily postponed until after hours, and relationships need constant tending. More equal measures of love and work sustain me, options that were not available to my mother.

Indeed, my mother "could have done some things." She earned her career, working hard in difficult times. Because she was one of only three women in a medical school class, there is a temptation to say she was obligated to continue, no matter what. But as this doctor's daughter, I benefited from her choices and her sacrifices. "From one to another," she passed on to me a legacy of competence and a courage tempered with love, a battered brown medical bag and a dictionary. I understand what I did not see before.

The Escape

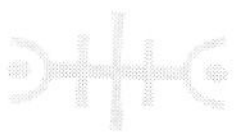

MANI RAJAGOPALAN, MD, DPM, DNB

It was going to be another routine assessment. The workload of psychiatrists had increased steadily ever since euthanasia was legalized several months ago. What started off as an occasional referral from a palliative care setting had gradually turned into a steady stream of requests from other departments as well.

The Euthanasia Specific Competency Assessment and Psychiatric Examination (ESCAPE) consisted of a structured questionnaire and mental state examination. Like most medical forms, it was several pages long and had to be completed in triplicate. I had been called to see a 31-year-old woman with secondary carcinoma in the brain from breast primary carcinoma. Basically, all I had to do was certify that the patient in question was not clinically depressed and was capable of making a decision. Although the legislation had been in effect for 8 months, many physicians and psychiatrists were unwilling to get involved, and it was left to a few of us who were progressive enough to consider euthanasia a viable option to do the assessments.

Having always believed that the right to die was as important as any other right, I had no qualms about being the psychiatrist on the Hospital Euthanasia Committee. Not that there was much competition for that position, anyway. To me, it was a small step from withdrawal of life support to assisting suicide in the terminally ill—both produced the same result, and I couldn't see what the fuss was all about. The proponents of the "Above all, do no harm" approach (the "Hippocratic" lobby) failed to accept that harm could just as easily be interpreted as letting someone suffer endlessly, with no relief in sight.

I reviewed the patient's case file and made a few notes. The paperwork from two independent physicians was complete. There was no doubt about the diagnosis; the condition was inoperable, and the patient's pain and distress were obvious. Progressive deterioration and increasing neurologic deficits were well documented by repeated assessments. She did not seem to have a significant psychiatric history. The nurses' reports described her as cheerful and cooperative despite her pain. She had been married for a short time, but her husband had died in a mining accident 3 years ago. She had no children. I could see that certifying this patient was going to be a mere formality.

I found her sitting up in bed, trying to change the channels on the television. She struggled to use the remote control, and the extent of her disability was apparent. Her features suggested that she was probably quite attractive once, but the wasting and hair loss made her look about two decades older than her 31 years. It was when she started to speak that I made the connection. I had known her many years ago in high school; I had even dated her a few times. We grew apart when I went away to medical school and had had no contact with each other since then. I could scarcely have imagined that I would meet her in this situation.

After the initial pleasantries and mutual expressions of surprise on both sides, we chatted for a while and caught up on all that had happened since we last met. For a few fleeting moments, we were two old friends meeting after many years. The moment passed, and we eventually got down to discussing her present condition. It wasn't easy for me to see her like this, but she was very clear about what she wanted to do, which made my job a little easier. She showed no evidence of depression. When I questioned her about her decision to die, she said, "Can you give me one good reason why I should go on living?" Quite frankly, I couldn't.

I promised to visit again the next day, and as I left, I added, "Since we know each other, I'll arrange for a second psychiatric opinion, just to be safe. After all, we don't want some hotshot lawyer from one of those radical anti-euthanasia groups holding us up on a technicality."

"I don't mind," she said. "As long as it's done quickly."

"I can see to that, " I replied. "And once that's completed, I'll forward the application to the Euthanasia Review Board. They hold fortnightly hearings in hospitals where there are requests. If the Board approves, we can go ahead with the procedure 48 hours later." She nodded in agreement.

At the nursing station, I noticed a small tremor as I tried to fill in the form. I hesitated. I had struggled to keep a lid on my emotions during the interview, but now they surfaced all at once. My signature on a form was the only thing she required to leave this world. It would also be the last thing she would ever need. Until today, I had had no problems with what I was doing, but this time, the gravity of my collective actions over the past few months started to take its toll. My last two patients had been a 72-year-old man with disseminated tumors and a 55-year-old woman with multiple sclerosis. It was one thing to certify and recommend people I had never seen before (and who were, at some unconscious level, probably less "real" to me) and another thing to send someone I knew down a path of no return. A series of questions passed through my mind. How does one go about certifying one's ex-girlfriend? What gave me the power to authoritatively state that someone was sane enough to commit what increasingly seemed to be an insane act? And isn't everyone someone's ex-girlfriend, someone's daughter, mother, or sister? If what I was doing was so right, how come it suddenly started to feel so wrong? Memories of high school came flooding in, and I left the ward rapidly.

Later that evening, I wrote a letter to the dean requesting that my name be taken off the panel of physicians on the Euthanasia Committee. I gave no reason except the usual "personal circumstances." To be professional is to act in the best interests of the patient. To be professional is to be detached, but how good is detachment when one is dealing with human beings? Does detachment automatically go hand in hand with what is best for the patient? I wrestled with these issues as I made my way home that winter evening, gentle snowflakes caressing my windshield.

Chained Smoker

DAVID S. SHIMM, MD

The man sat in the examination chair as the physician talked to him. He could feel the sunlight coming through the window, warming his face. If he looked toward the window, the sunlight dazzled him, and when he turned his face away, it still painted the periphery of his vision with a haze of red. To his right, he could see where pieces of plaster had fallen out of the walls and ceiling of the small examination room, leaving specks and blotches of white drywall showing through the dull, lime-green paint. Farther to his right, he could see the metal instrument table. Probes and mirrors lay in the half-opened drawers, neatly arranged, menacing. On the table, an alcohol lamp faintly flickered with a pungent smell that reminded him of his first, frightening encounters with his childhood physician. He felt a twinge of nausea.

Although in his fifties, he looked like an old man. His face was tanned and wrinkled, and his cheeks and lips were sunken because he had no teeth to fill them out. His gaunt temples emphasized his dark, sunken eyes. He had a full head of oily, unkempt black hair that was peppered with gray. On his hands and forearms were several crude tattoos in faded ballpoint pen. One spelled his ex-wife's name, and another represented the torso of a nude, headless woman. Various cellmates had etched these tattoos as they passed monotonous hours in the county jail for petty offenses: fighting, public drunkenness, driving under the influence of alcohol. The index and middle fingers of both his hands were stained brown, one of the stigmata of his years of smoking. His hands were calloused, and there were deep cracks in his skin around his knuckles. His left ring finger was missing above the first joint. His life had been rough, and his body bore the scars of the abuse that had been done to him by others and by himself.

He had gone to the physician because of pain in his tongue and an ache in his ear when he swallowed. Although he initially brushed it off, the pain became so bad when he swallowed that he had stopped eating; he had already lost 15 pounds. He had seen this physician for the first time 2 days earlier. The physician spent an eternity asking questions and examining him. After he finished, he told the man that he probably had a malignant tumor in his tongue, but he needed to do a biopsy to be sure.

A needle jabbed, and then he felt a deep, painful ache that faded into numbness as the anesthetic was injected. He gripped the armrests tightly, mouth open wide, eyes closed and tearing. Although the biopsy itself did not hurt, the feeling of tissue being torn from his tongue without pain was almost worse than the pain of the injection. After that, he was aware of the metallic taste of blood and, later, a dull ache as the anesthetic wore off.

"The results of your biopsy are back," said the physician.

The man waited for him to continue.

The physician hesitated. "I'm sorry, it doesn't look good. You have a malignant tumor in your tongue."

"How did it get there?" asked the man.

"Almost certainly from smoking. It's rare to see these tumors in people who don't smoke, and your drinking probably contributed as well."

"What are my chances?"

"That depends," said the physician. "There are two ways of treating this. The first way is to operate. We would have to take out most of your tongue, part of your jaw, and the lymph glands in your neck.

It's a fairly big operation, and you'd probably be in the hospital for a couple of weeks, maybe even a month if you had problems healing. The other way would be to treat you with chemotherapy and radiation. With those, you'd probably have some nausea, you'd have a bad sore throat, and afterwards your mouth would be permanently dry. With either treatment, you've got about a 50-50 chance."

"No good choices, I guess. What if I do nothing?"

The physician paused before responding. "Well, the tumor would continue to grow."

"And how would it kill me?"

"Well, in this location, it would either grow big enough to choke off your airway or keep you from swallowing, or it would eat into a blood vessel and you'd bleed to death. Not very gentle ways to go. I really wouldn't recommend doing nothing. There's still a reasonable chance of curing this tumor." The two stared at one another for a moment before the physician continued. "Another thing . . . it's really important for you to quit smoking. I know it's hard, but if you do, you'll tolerate the treatment better, and you'll be less likely to get another kind of cancer later."

The man sat staring at the wall, focusing on one of the spots of drywall showing through. He felt numb, just as he did whenever his foot fell asleep, a numbness that took his strength away. But this time it wasn't his foot: It was his mind and his soul that were numb. He shook his head to try to clear his thinking.

"How much time do I have to decide?"

"You really need to make a decision in the next few days," answered the physician. "Time isn't on your side, but this is an important decision, and you need to feel comfortable with your choice. Let's make an appointment for you to come in and talk right after lunch, the day after tomorrow."

The man nodded and sat in the chair for a few more moments. He put his hands on his knees and pushed himself upright. He walked out of the examination room and down the hall to the exit. As he pushed through the door, the sunlight was so bright that he had to squint. After a second, his eyes adjusted, and he could see the mountains in the background, behind the trees. A few feet away, next to the doorway, there was a bench.

The man sat down, looked again at the mountains, and took a deep breath. He swallowed, and there was the pain again, stabbing into his ear. He reached into his shirt pocket and took out his pack of cigarettes. Holding the pack between thumb and forefinger, he examined it. He closed his hand around the pack to crush it but then stopped. He removed a cigarette, put it in his mouth, and pulled a nearly empty book of matches from between the cardboard and the cellophane. Striking a match, he lit the cigarette, took it from his mouth, and held it to the stoma he had breathed through since he had lost his larynx to cancer. He inhaled deeply.

The Coding Audit

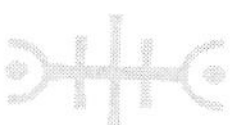

JOAN SUMKIN, MD

You need two out of three components to code a 99213. Understand, this has nothing to do with the quality of medical care. The reality is that HCFA [the Health Care Financing Administration] will reclaim fees paid for inaccurate coding."

A pile of my audited charts was arranged in front of the coding consultant. Next to her sat our billing specialist. It was 8:30 on a Thursday morning, in the middle of the half hour that I usually reserve to think, dictate letters, read about my difficult cases, and perform the myriad tasks that pile up by the end of the week. I understood that our group had actually requested this review. The mastery of evaluation and management codes was as much a requirement for medicine in the 1990s as board certification. I had mentally prepared myself (or so I had thought) to handle this critique of my billing practices.

What I didn't expect was the unbidden escalation of my annoyance as we began the scripted process. The coding consultant started with my raw data. Twelve of 22 charts were coded properly; just 55% correct. My scalp started to prickle. The consultant explained that the inconsistencies were errors of either upcoding or downcoding. Since I had always thought that upcoding (charging more than supported by documentation) was the egregious error, my chief concern was the two charts that apparently did not pass muster in this category.

The consultant leveled me with her look. "*Any* error in coding can potentially cause penalty," she said. "Those five cases that you undercoded are a red flag to HCFA. They signal that you don't know how to code, and that can prompt a full audit. And then payments can be reclaimed. . . ." She droned on in her imperious tone. And I started to smolder.

I was angry that billing issues could even evoke in me that kind of emotion. With all of the ups and downs of training and clinical practice, I had gained a wider perspective and a cooler temperament than I had had in medical school days. Control of feelings was an element of my job. This sense of aggravation was, frankly, silly. But it was there! The spark ignited and I felt the fire flare.

"This doesn't take into account the time I spent explaining the issues to the patient, calling the family, calling the specialist, and making special arrangements, or the time spent thinking, feeling, caring. . . ." The consultant stopped me halfway through my diatribe.

"What you do doesn't matter," she said patiently. "If you don't document it correctly, you don't get reimbursed and you could get fined."

There it was. Bureaucratic arrogance was the crux of my frustration. The dissection of the medical encounter had become so detailed that actual patient interaction was now secondary to fleshing out the chart for HCFA.

I wanted to say all this, but instead I kept silent. Emotional pyrotechnics would be wasted on them while consuming me. The coding consultant and the billing specialist were getting uncomfortable. They truly had no context for understanding.

By the time the meeting ended, I was 10 minutes late for my 9:00 patient. I found it difficult to concentrate during the consultation. The elements of coding hounded me. Did I get enough review of systems for a 99214? How about pertinent PFSH (Past, Family, and Social History)? How complex was her problem, anyway? Was it moderately complex or highly complex? By whose standards?

Later that day, between appointments, I checked messages and mail. There was a letter addressed to me with PERSONAL stamped on the front. I opened it and found a notecard decorated with flowers and headlined "Thinking of You." It was carefully typed.

> Dear Dr. Sumkin,
>
> How are you? I hope you don't mind me writing you a note. It was very good to see you in the parking lot a week ago. I miss you sometimes. We have been through a lot together. You were always there for me. I know I can't waste your time and the state's money but sometimes I would just like to set and talk a bit. I could always tell you how I was feeling inside and out and you never put me down. You never made me feel like I was worthless or dumb. Thank you.

As the letter went on, the heat dissipated. I entered the next exam room . . . a doctor.

Heartsick

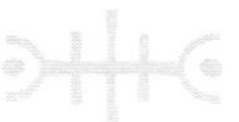

JULIA E. McMURRAY, MD

"Hello, Miz Lucy," I would say as my father led me into the patient exam room. Miz Lucy, a diminutive retired schoolteacher, would be sitting in the chair, gussied up to the nines, with gnarled hands and feet shod in heavy stockings and thick orthopedic shoes. My father, a general internist in a small southern town, would have me touch her swollen hands as he injected the gold that would help her pain. She would exclaim about my growth, my successes in school, and would mention how the good doctor had saved her life more than once. Later, she would drive by our house in her ancient green Cadillac to make sure that he was home in case she needed him or to drop off her special cookies. At Christmas time, our kitchen counter was always covered with cakes, pies, or crocheted afghans made by grateful patients like Miz Lucy.

I remember making a house call with my father on a wintery Sunday afternoon. We drove up to a small house in which a sad, weathered-looking man with slumped shoulders sat in a wheelchair.

"Arthur," my dad would say as he took off his coat and opened up his massive black bag, "how are you?" And the murmuring would start. I would sit on the sofa in the quiet, empty house and watch as my father talked with Arthur. Later, on the drive home, my father would tell me how, as a young man, Arthur had dived into a quarry pond and severed his spinal cord.

And then there was Margaret. Struck down by polio at the age of 9 in a tiny farm town up in the county, Margaret survived in an iron lung; her brother had died. Her mother had cared for her all her life, even moving to a major university town long enough to help Margaret get a college degree. Margaret, only her head visible while her wasted body was encased in the huge tubular machine, would ask me about my latest book while my father inspected her mother's diabetic foot ulcer or assessed Margaret's recurrent parotitis. Margaret's mother eventually developed dementia and, before she died, cursed the daughter whom she had cared for all her life. To this day, my now-retired father still visits weekly, to discuss books, to bring medicines. I still visit at Christmas with my father, taking my children along with me.

These memories are my most enduring and are at the heart of why I became a physician. Now, after nearly 15 years in various practices, having raised my children and finally settled down in a group practice of dedicated, like-minded colleagues, I am glad that I kept the name that connects me to my father and to his legacy of doctoring. I have a dream and the guts to begin to fulfill it, a dream of building a practice with my Miz Lucys and Arthurs and Margarets. My dream is to provide superb medical care as I get to know them over time, to be their physician in my sense of the word, and to grow old with them.

But managed care is threatening that dream. "Growth and profit," the business executive writes on the blackboard as he explains that the practice of assigning patients to individual physicians has been abolished and that patients may sign up with any physician, regardless of known waits for routine or urgent care.

"For a panel size of 4000, we will pay you *x* more dollars in salary than for the current 2000 patients you are managing," he intones. Our protests are not acknowledged, and our reluctance to add more patients to already jammed practices is seen as "slothful and needy."

As the months go by, my established patients become more unhappy as it becomes more difficult for them to see me. My new patients are enraged at the more than 3 months' wait for a physical. They feel betrayed by the slick advertisements and come-ons. In the office, they sit with lists written on the backs of envelopes to remind them to discuss their headaches, constipation, elevated cholesterol and hormone levels. There just doesn't seem to be enough time for them to begin to trust me, nor for me to understand the person behind the list. I dread looking at my daily schedule and long for the short, uncomplicated medical encounter. My face no longer lights up in anticipation of opening the handwritten letter in my mailbox. Nowadays, these are much less likely to be testimonies to my care and much more likely to be complaints about the referral, the waits, or the most recent visit.

My Middle Eastern patient comes to see me. As always, she wears traditional Muslim clothing, her round face peering out of her headdress. Widowed and alone, she is suing her employer for sexual harassment in a long, arduous battle that will determine whether she can continue in the research career that she loves. I have been so impressed with the pluck and courage of this shy, lonely woman fighting to survive in a radically different culture. Our visits usually move quickly through the hypertension and the knee pain to the real reason for her visit: my support, my affirmation, and my reassurance that she will be all right. I see the hurt in her eyes as I am pushed for time one day and brusquely cut short our discussion.

A new patient calls me on the phone. She has menstrual irregularities, insomnia, and mood swings, and the suspicion that she is menopausal has added the stress of a major life transition to her already present difficulties. The wait for an appointment with me is unacceptably long to her. Although I have never seen her, on paper I am already her physician, and she is angry and irritated. I call her back, having already added extra patients to my session that day. Sitting in my office with my elbows on a stack of charts that all bear notes asking me to call patients, I am overwhelmed and vaguely realize that our conversation hasn't gone well. Many weeks later, when we finally meet, my new patient forcefully condemns my lack of compassion on the phone and is uninterested in both my abject apologies and my explanations about "HMO panel sizes" and "time pressures." I know that she has labeled me arrogant and insensitive, and the sense of failure on my part is enormous. Although I spend time rationalizing and working through the experience, her diatribe against me remains one of the most painful moments in my 15 years of doctoring.

I begin to feel as if I am in a war. I speak out at meetings but feel small and unheard. I want to ask the managers and my bosses, "Where do you get your health care, and if your elderly mother is ill, do you want her to see the kind of physician you are attempting to create?" It is the practitioners and patients who will reap what these corporatized leaders have sown.

What about my dream? It has nothing to do with income, with status, or with having built a more cost-effective medical machine but is about the deep satisfaction that my interpersonal relationships and skills with my patients over the years will bring. Above all else, the physician–patient relationship must be preserved. I do not see this happening, despite my dedication to it and my efforts to sound an alarm and rouse my colleagues to action. I feel a helplessness as I face this inexorable attack. I am simply heartsick.

Annual Meeting: Perspectives

KEITH WRENN, MD

He was early. No one besides the audiovisual guy was there. It was a big room with several hundred uncomfortable chairs, all too close together. He chose one on the aisle about halfway back. The temperature was just a little too chilly. As he sat down, he sighed with relief.

He was a general internist in a town with one red light. Getting here had been frustrating. First, he'd spent the last 2 weeks working extra hard, trying to keep his chronically ill patients doing as well as they could, out of the hospital. The last week had been a blur of activity, attempting to get his census of inpatients down. Then there had been the inevitable last-minute crises: chest pain, fever, a dead leg. It was never a tidy process.

His wife was upset because of the extra-long days and because he'd been so preoccupied recently. Now he'd be out of town for 5 days. She didn't get to go to meetings, and she didn't buy his line that the meetings were really work. He was going to miss one son's basketball game and the other's Boy Scout Jamboree. His partner was not too happy either: more calls, more patients, and less sleep.

Then there was the cost: plane tickets, hotel, meals, and all the other incidentals. Every year it was more than a thousand dollars. Although it was tax deductible, it was still a major outlay, more than 1% of his annual income.

Nevertheless, he was happy to be here. This was his major continuing medical education effort for the year. He loved to hear about new things or to have the old things he did justified by experts. He tried to keep up with his journals, but it was a losing battle. He just didn't have protected time.

He saw old friends from training and caught up on other people from his past. The flying and staying in a hotel always seemed exciting to him, and being alone, away from his telephone, was very relaxing. He always felt rejuvenated when he returned to his practice.

* * * *

She was early. The audiovisual guy was up on the stage testing the microphone and the pointer. There was already someone in the audience, hands behind his head, staring at the ceiling. She hated to be this early, but she couldn't help herself. Despite having given some version of this talk half a dozen times, she still got anxious beforehand. She was an academic, chief of her division, a scientist of some renown. She had a lot to manage: grants, faculty, residents, and students. Getting here had been hectic. There was an important committee meeting that needed to be rescheduled. She had a grant to review and a couple of papers to edit. Then her research fellow had a problem with the cell cultures. And of course, there were always some last-minute slides for her secretary to prepare.

She wasn't on service this month, so there weren't any loose ends to tie up on the wards. Thank God she'd be able to fly out tonight and get back home. Her husband didn't mind the overnight trips. He used to come with her, but she traveled too much now. Thank God she didn't have to pay for these trips either. She didn't enjoy flying much anymore or hotels, but at least the college paid for all of this. Her income wasn't that great.

She was grateful that she didn't have to depend on these big meetings to keep up, that she could walk down the hall to hear a lecture every day at the university. She didn't have the time anymore for a meeting like this.

Although this talk was a distraction, it would at least be over in an hour and a half. These kinds of talks were good for her reputation and for the reputation of her department and institution. This talk, in particular, had been well received in the past. Reading the evaluations made her feel worthwhile.

She enjoyed seeing some old friends, residents, and students. Now, however, there were faces she couldn't remember, times when she feigned recognition. And there were others whom she'd just as soon not see.

As the speaker walked toward the podium, she passed the general internist. They both nodded, and each felt a twinge of envy.

Chronic Active Adolescence

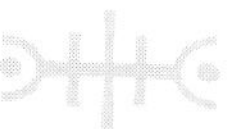

CHRISTOPHER M. CALLAHAN, MD

It was 1980. Michael was sitting in his dormitory room making the final summary sheet for 7 weeks of classroom notes. The notes he had scribbled in haste had been rewritten in a beautiful cursive and then exposed to the scrutiny of yellow and pink fluorescent highlighters. The summary sheet itself was coded in the ink of four different pens. The distilled facts that made it onto his final summary sheet held the key to a final grade of "A." Michael knew that if he transposed this information onto his brain he would indeed perform heroically on the examination. He had perfected the process in 8 years of grade school, 4 years of high school, 4 years of college, and his first year of medical school.

His roommate, Kevin, snuck up behind him and slapped headphones blaring rock and roll onto Michael's ears. Kevin was wearing a towel and dripping the remnants of his shower on Michael's final summary sheet. Michael quickly saved the work from further defacement and shook the headphones off with a jerk of his head.

"Goin' to the party tonight, Ace? I heard Karin's gonna be there," Kevin asked, dancing badly beside Michael's desk.

Michael smiled. He liked his identity of "the Ace." Michael wasn't looking at Kevin. He spoke to a poster of Krebs' cycle that he had hanging over his desk.

"No, I'm not goin'. I've still got some studying to do. I haven't even started on my anatomy summary sheet yet."

"Jeez, give it a rest, Mike. Everyone is takin' the night off."

"Maybe some other time. Tell Karin I said 'hi'."

"Yeah . . . right, Mike. 'Karin, Michael says hi.' I'm sure she'll be impressed."

Michael believed that Karin would be impressed. Impressed by his dedication, his focus, his mission, his martyrdom. Everyone else was. Throughout his schooling, everyone had told him so. He was the Ace.

Michael knew the difference between Kevin and himself—Kevin had chosen to keep one foot in the world outside of medical training. Kevin was not a true follower of Time Fragmentation Theory. Disciples of this theory found efficiency in overtly dividing their near future into digestible chunks of time for the purpose of focusing on the next big hurdle. Time might be fragmented into the number of days left before the big test, the end of the semester, or graduation. The individual thereby voluntarily placed his or her life on deferment for the purpose of clearing the next hurdle. Time Fragmentation Theory was delayed gratification for professionals. The true effect of this Time Fragmentation Theory was to suspend the individual's awareness that he or she was actually currently living a life. One day Michael would realize that Time Fragmentation Theory was a delusion. He would seek compensation for his lost time. He would feel victimized.

It was 1985. Michael had Christmas off. He needed the break from his residency. He complained half-heartedly that he shouldn't leave the hospital because he might miss some good cases. What an Ace, his colleagues beamed. Most of his family was home for Christmas. His mother remarked that he looked terrible. He hadn't had time to eat or exercise, he explained. If he wanted to land that fellowship, he had to make the grade. Michael's dad looked old. He seemed to have aged since Michael had gone away to college almost 10 years earlier. His little brother, Tom, and Tom's wife and daughter were also home for the holidays. Tom was a vice president at his company now. He owned a nice home, and he and his wife were active in the community. Tom and his wife played golf on weekends with friends from church. They had just gotten back from a vacation in Europe. Tom and Dad seemed to have a lot to talk about: raising a family, running a business, his mother's health. His mother's health? Why didn't he know about Mom's health? He was the doctor.

"Oh, we didn't want to worry you about that. How's school going, Ace?"

Michael escaped the discomfort of his parents' home to meet two of his buddies from high school for a drink. They had whole lives already: marriages, births, careers, travel, relationships, and responsibilities in the world.

"When are you going to finish school and get a job?" they asked.

Michael began to think about his prolonged sophomoric status. His teens and early twenties had been spent cramming for the big test. Now, in his late twenties, he still had someone else determining his schedule—when to report for rounds, when to go home for the evening. He had to live with supervision and evaluations, patients wanting to talk to the "real doctor," nurses questioning his judgment, and attending physicians highlighting his inadequacies. Just a few more years now, he rationalized, and his apprenticeship would be over. When he got back from his Christmas break, he borrowed money to buy a new sports car and asked one of the ICU nurses for a date that Saturday night. She was married, she said incredulously, waving her ring finger. He ended up having to work late on Saturday anyway. His new car got a dent sitting in the parking lot. Someone would pay for this, he fumed. He began to feel victimized.

It was 1990. Michael was on staff. He had cleared his last hurdle, and his life was officially off deferment at the age of 32. Bring on adulthood and all of its rewards! He had a busy clinic and kept track of appointments, procedures, and patient data in his new electronic personal organizer. He had a new car and a new house. Michael finally made the kind of money he felt he earned. As the months passed, the car sat in the parking lot, where it collected rust while he spent his days and evenings in the clinic and the hospital. He hadn't made any new friends and he didn't have many old ones left. His father had died recently. He hadn't identified the perfect woman yet. He got a bad grade on his 6-month physician profile. He was an outlier on six of 12 indicators. Two nurses complained that he was arrogant and egotistical. Four patients reported that he was obnoxious and paternalistic. He had a fight with the semiretired former chief-of-staff in front of a patient. The former chief-of-staff reported that Michael was a problem.

They were all fools, Michael thought to himself as he circled the wagons, they were lucky to have a talented young physician like him on staff. He had been victimized! Over the coming months, his victimization gave rise to anger and frustration and finally to disillusionment. Michael wallowed in self-pity for a year or so, and then went to visit his old roommate, Kevin. Kevin sat behind a desk loaded with charts, regulations, practice guidelines, journals, correspondence, stale coffee, and half his lunch. Michael related his misfortune. Kevin understood completely; he had had the same affliction, but he had never given up his foothold in the world outside medical training.

"You're suffering from chronic active adolescence," Kevin explained. "We've all been through the same thing. We flourished for years in a system where we based our identity on standardized examinations. We learned to thrive in the role of adolescent, and some of us even learned to put adult relationships and responsibilities on hold for over a decade in a curious attempt to focus on our training. When you finish your training, you're supposed to begin functioning in the world that you put on deferment sometime back in high school. The sad part is that you soon realize that the world wasn't really on hold at all, and then you feel victimized when people don't salute your perceived sacrifices. Frankly, nobody cares that you were the top of your class and . . ."

"Fine, so you're telling me to grow up," Michael responded impatiently. "How will I know when I'm cured?"

"When you stop worrying about grades and start embracing relationships. When you stop dwelling on what you gave up to become a physician and start focusing on what you get back. When you feel humbled rather than victimized."

The Making of a Public Health Physician

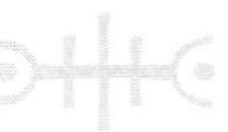

KATHLEEN F. GENSHEIMER, MD, MPH

My husband and I got married the week before match day during our fourth year of medical school. Upon our return from our wedding trip, we were very relieved to discover that we would not only be located within the same city but would also be doing our internships at the same institution. I was starting a postgraduate training program in pediatrics; my husband was doing a rotating internship before going onto a residency in ophthalmology. Unfortunately, our on-call schedule never seemed to coincide; hence, we spent that year following a discordant cycle of one night on, the next night totally exhausted, and the third night trying to gain the physical and emotional stamina to face the following night's trials. Our crock pot worked overtime creating many a dinner. Whoever was home on a given evening hauled its overcooked contents through the streets of Philadelphia to eventually share with the other in some dismal on-call room. For me, the highlight of the year was contracting pertussis and being banned from on-call duty in the neonatal intensive care nursery for several nights. And acquiring hepatitis B from a needle-stick exposure gave my husband the time to reupholster our couch and chairs.

Late in the academic year, I decided to seek a pediatric training program elsewhere in the city. Unfortunately, no position was available, and I was told that I would have to wait another year for an opening. Because our undergraduate loans required monthly payments, I had no choice but to find other work in the interim. I stumbled onto a public health residency training program offered by the New Jersey Department of Health.

The regular hours offered by this residency allowed us to start a family. We soon began the frantic search for quality, affordable child care and worried endlessly about our infant daughter while we were at work. Our life seemed torn apart, our loyalties divided, as we attempted to be with our daughter as much as possible while simultaneously trying to meet the academic demands placed on us. I vividly recall my daughter crying inconsolably for the first 3 months of her life. In retrospect, I believe that she did not suffer from colic; I'm convinced that she suffered from having an overly anxious mother. My fears that all I was doing was wrong were fueled by the neighbors' never-ending, freely dispensed advice. Compounding those fears was the tremendous sense of guilt I suffered every morning as I left the crying baby in the care of one in a long line of ever-changing child-care providers. Even my efforts to calm her while nursing must have been thwarted by the production of adrenaline-rich milk.

As I eased more comfortably into motherhood, I was able to concentrate on my residency and I found myself more enthusiastic about the work than I had initially believed possible. I became especially interested in the public health applications of epidemiology and applied to the Epidemic Intelligence Service (EIS) program at the Centers for Disease Control (CDC). At that point, I was a mother of a 15-month-old child and in the early stages of pregnancy with baby number two. This scenario created concern on the part of CDC about my suitability for acceptance to the incoming EIS class. A pregnant EIS recruit was an unknown entity, and as I interviewed for one potential assignment after the next, I could feel the cool reception as I entered each office. But the health officer in Maine was not afraid to give a pregnant recruit a chance, so an assignment to Maine was the ultimate outcome of the EIS match.

We arrived in Maine in early August, greeted by the rain, fog, and chill of what we were to learn was a typical summer day. I started work the following Monday, leaving my husband as temporary child-care provider. The moment I returned home at the end of the day, he would disappear into the far corners of our rambling 1796 house to renovate what was to become his office while I nursed my infant son and simultaneously balanced my young daughter on my lap. Our weekends were filled with looking for a suitable child-care provider, unpacking, and settling the family into the new home.

I had been continually instructed by my CDC mentors to go out and "find those outbreaks!" Find them I did, even on holidays and weekends. Trying to be a true shoe-leather epidemiologist, I had no recourse but to take the two young children with me on outbreak investigations after hours, when child care was especially difficult to arrange. A salmonellosis investigation over the July 4th weekend was especially memorable. I locked the two kids in the vehicle (fortunately, no one reported me to the Child Protective Unit of the Maine Department of Human Services) while I interviewed the manager, staff, and food handlers of a national fast-food chain restaurant. During the course of the investigation, I confiscated suspect food for laboratory testing and stashed it in the car. Later, while I was inside the local hospital reviewing the emergency department log for potential cases of salmonellosis, the two kids happily munched on the confiscated food. After thoroughly berating the poor kids for "eating Mommy's work," I rushed back to the implicated restaurant for more specimens. Neither of the kids became symptomatic, so I was able to enroll them as controls in my study.

Realizing that my training was still not adequate for a practicing epidemiologist and taking advantage of a depressed economy in Maine (where members of the state government workforce were encouraged to resign, retire early, or take an unpaid leave of absence), I decided to return to school to pursue a master's degree in public health. Now with four children, ages 11, 9, 7, and 4, I moved to Boston, leaving my husband behind to maintain his practice and financially support my academic pursuits. I found the return to the classroom gratifying and fulfilling. It also put me on an equal footing with my school-age children: We spent evenings commiserating over extensive reading assignments, unfair examinations, and unrealistic teachers. Long after I'd put them to bed, I sat in front of my newly acquired computer, struggling to meet assignment deadlines. Our weekends were spent commuting back and forth to Maine so that my 9-year-old could fill his lungs "with that clean Maine air." With the end of school and my return to work in Maine, my reward for pursuing further training was a cut in salary and increased responsibilities, the typical scenario for a public health practitioner.

My career as an epidemiologist has been a family affair. The kids have been influenced by my work over the years, as demonstrated by my son's show-and-tell in kindergarten, when he apparently provided an all-too-vivid description of *Escherichia coli* O157:H7 infection and bad hamburger. My career choices have been influenced by the various stages in development of my marriage and family; as a result, I have had the flexibility to respond to the needs of a growing family. My personal and professional life is very fulfilling and richer because my husband and four children have provided me with a broader perspective on life. My needs as a working mother have guided my public health efforts in Maine; hence, I have become involved in such issues as infectious disease threats in child-care settings, injury control, and promoting a safer food supply. I like to think that my work as a public health practitioner has been enhanced by my training and by the personal events, opportunities, and chance occurrences that have culminated in a rewarding career.

Communion

RICHARD B. WEINBERG, MD

I am not an intimidating person, but I found my last patient of the day huddled in the corner of the examining room, as if awaiting an executioner. She was in her mid-twenties, and she clutched a sheaf of medical records against her chest like a shield. She had made the appointment to our clinic herself. The face sheet on her chart said "chronic abdominal pain."

I introduced myself, sat down, and began to take her history. She had had severe abdominal pain since her mid-teens, but her description of the pain was so vague that no specific diagnosis sprang to mind. And her records disclosed that other physicians had fared no better: She had been seen at every major gastroenterology clinic in town, had gone through all the tests, and had tried all the medicines. What, I asked myself, kept her trudging from doctor to doctor on this medical odyssey? And what could I possibly do for her?

As I questioned her, I studied her with growing fascination. She was anxious and withdrawn, but nonetheless she projected a desperate courage, like a cornered animal making a defiant last stand. She kept her gaze directed downward, but every now and then I caught her staring at me intensely, as if searching for something. She wore a drab, bulky sweater and oversized bluejeans, and her unkempt hair fell over her eyes. It struck me that she deliberately had done everything possible to obscure the fact that she was a very attractive young woman.

She seemed so uncomfortable talking about herself that I moved on to inquire about her family history. Her parents had emigrated from Italy. Her mother had died when she was a young girl and, although she was not the oldest child, it had fallen to her to play the role of mother to her five siblings. She was a devout Catholic, who, like her mother, attended mass every morning. "But I don't take communion," she added. Her father was a baker and through years of hard work now owned his own bakery, which she managed.

Now, cooking is my hobby, but baking is one culinary skill I have never mastered. So I was always on the lookout for good bakeries, for they are not easy to come by. I asked where her bakery was and if they made French pastries, one of my weaknesses. They did. "Are they as good as the French Gourmet Bakery's?" I asked, mentioning the name of a popular bakery near the medical center. "I'm addicted to their Napoleons."

For the first time her eyes came alive. "I wouldn't feed pastries from the French Gourmet to my cat," she retorted. "The French learned all they know about baking from the Italians," she informed me with an artisan's pride. "It's not as easy to make Napoleons as it looks—it's very tricky," she said, with a tone of voice that implied that she knew the secret, but she was certainly not about to tell me. Her passionate outburst took me by surprise, but it faded away as quickly as it had appeared. The remainder of the interview was monosyllabic.

Her physical examination was entirely normal. I told her that I thought she most likely had a severe form of irritable bowel syndrome. She listened carefully, but said nothing. I prescribed a bland diet and the one antispasmodic she had yet to try, and asked her to return in one month. I was not optimistic.

I really didn't expect to see her again, but she reappeared the next week. As before, she sat silently in the examining room, and responded to my questions with terse replies. Because she had become so animated talking about the bakery the week before, and because baking seemed to be the only point of contact I had established with this otherwise withdrawn young woman, I spent most of the visit asking her about Italian pastries: which ones sold on which holidays, what kind of yeast worked best, the recipes her father had brought from Italy. She was very knowledgeable. She didn't mention anything about abdominal pain. I made another return appointment for a month later.

Again she returned the next week. This time she seemed a bit more at ease, but I noted the dark rings under her eyes. "Are you sleeping well?" I inquired.

"No."

"Why?"

"Because I have a nightmare."

"A nightmare? The same nightmare every night?"

"Yes."

"Can you tell me about it?" She was silent for some time, and then took a deep breath, as if she had made a decision. Then, in a barely audible monotone, she described her dream: She is running, because she must get to confession before the priest leaves. But when she enters the church it is empty, dark, cold. She calls out, but there is no answer. Suddenly, unseen acolytes seize her and drag her to the altar. Her head is pulled back and holy water is forced down her throat to drown her screams. She struggles to raise her head and sees a procession of hooded priests holding long candles headed up the aisle toward her. I shuddered as I listened to her; the implication of the lurid imagery was inescapable.

"Were you ever sexually assaulted?" I asked gently.

"Yes."

"When?"

"When I was fourteen." She was breathing now in short, rapid gasps. I didn't know whether to continue or not. Her eyes said yes.

"What happened?" With great effort she told me. She had been raped by her oldest sister's boyfriend. He had come to the bakery late at night in search of her sister, but had found her instead. "There's nothing dirty he didn't do to me," she sobbed, and now unstoppable, she poured out the grim details of her ordeal.

"You never reported it?"

"No."

"You never told anyone?" She looked up at me with an imploring face. "How could I tell anyone . . . it would kill my father and destroy my family," she wept. "You're the only person I've ever told."

I felt completely out of my depth. I consoled her as best I could and, when her sobbing had subsided, I gently suggested a referral to a psychiatrist or rape counselor. I'm a gastroenterologist, I told her, this is not my area of expertise. I had neither the knowledge nor the experience to help her, I explained. But she adamantly refused to consider a referral to anyone else. She didn't trust them. I then understood that, having unearthed her dark secret, I had become responsible for her care.

So I scheduled weekly visits late in the day so she could talk as long as she wanted. I mostly listened. After the rape she had felt soiled and defiled, and inexplicably had felt a powerful need to be punished further for her "sin." She could no longer take communion. For weeks after her assault she could not eat. But then, insidiously, she fell into a ritual of penitence: She would sneak into the bakery late at night and stuff herself with pastries, then purge herself, and repeat the process until her stomach ached and she was exhausted. She was helpless to stop, for her bingeing ritual expiated her guilt and shame, albeit only briefly.

She seemed to derive great strength from the visits. When discussion became difficult, we talked about baking. I spent many evenings in the medical library reading as much as I could about rape and subsequent eating disorders. There was not much written, and after a while it seemed that I was learning more from my patient than from the clinical journals. Still uneasy with my unaccustomed role, I discussed her case with a colleague in the psychiatry department.

"Is she comfortable talking with you?" he asked.

"Yes."

"Does she seem to be getting better?"

"I think so."

"Then you're doing just as well as we could," he declared.

The visits continued and, as the months passed, I noted subtle but unmistakable changes: Her anxious look vanished and she began to smile; she gained some weight and remarked that she thought it made her look better; a touch of makeup appeared; she came to the clinic with a new hairstyle; she informed me that she had returned to school part-time and had received her high school diploma. She announced that she was taking communion again. Her visits came at longer and longer intervals.

I hadn't seen her for 3 months, when she appeared just as I was about to leave the clinic. At first I didn't recognize her, such was the extent of her transformation. She was vibrant, alive. And she looked beautiful—elegantly attired as if for a night on the town. I realized she had dressed up for me. I also sensed that something was completed, that this was a leave-taking. We sat down in the empty waiting room.

"I'm quitting the bakery," she told me. "I'm going to travel to Italy this summer, and when I get back I'm going to start college full-time. I wanted to see you before I left so I could bring you these," she said, handing me a white cardboard box, carefully tied with a bright ribbon. "Should I open it now?" I asked. She nodded.

Inside the box, neatly resting on individual doilies, were six perfect Napoleons, the pastry puffed high, the fondant a smooth glassy sheet, the chocolate chevrons meticulously aligned. "My father usually makes these, but he sometimes doesn't get it just right. I made these myself just for you," she said. I smiled and thanked her for her kindness. We talked a bit about her forthcoming trip. Then she stood to go.

"Thank you for believing in me," she said.

"I should say the same," I replied.

A thin film of tears shone in her eyes. She leaned toward me and kissed my cheek. "Goodbye," she whispered, then whirled down the hall to the elevator. Just as the doors opened, she turned back and flashed me a radiant smile that warmed me like the sun. "Don't eat them all at once," she said with a mischievous twinkle in her eye.

"It's not healthy, you know."

"A doctor doesn't choose his patients," the grey-haired professor who taught me physical diagnosis would say. "It is the patient who chooses the doctor." I had been chosen to receive a gift of trust, and of all the gifts I had ever received, none seemed as precious. That afternoon, I left the clinic feeling exhilarated and full of love for my profession. That evening, after dinner, I opened my present and partook of the communion from the baker's daughter.

Trying To Let Go

DAVID J. COSTIGAN, MD

Just the other day, I was in an intensive care unit in St. Louis, Missouri, evaluating a patient for a gastrostomy tube. Apparently, the patient had suffered an in-hospital cardiac arrest. The nurse began to give me more of the details. "After a prolonged, 1- to 2-hour code. . . ." Then it happened again: My mind began to wander.

It was 20 years ago in Philadelphia. I was a second-year resident in internal medicine, doing my training in a small community hospital affiliated with one of the area universities. I was only 28 years old. I had just lain down to rest after another long night putting out medical fires. Suddenly, I was awakened by a code blue in the emergency room. It was 6:00 A.M., and I raced to the point of contact. I imagined another terminally ill, elderly, unsalvageable patient who did not need resuscitation at all. I had seen so many cases in which our efforts were useless and frustrating. This case was different.

I soon met a beautiful 16-year-old girl who was in full cardiopulmonary arrest. I quickly learned that 8 hours earlier, this girl had come into the emergency room reporting shortness of breath and was discharged with the diagnosis of hyperventilation and anxiety. An arterial blood gas had been obtained, but for some unknown reason the patient was discharged before the laboratory report, which showed a

PO_2 of 50 mm Hg, was completed.

None of this made sense to me. How could the staff have sent her home before the blood gas results came back? How could they not have called her immediately after seeing such abnormal results? However it had happened, someone had decided not to call her back right away. That call was to wait until the morning.

She came back to the hospital in full arrest from a pulmonary embolus. She was in electromechanical dissociation. She was not responding to all routine measures. We did not have streptokinase. A thoracic surgeon was not in the hospital and was probably 30 to 45 minutes away. None of us knew how to open her chest. Time was slipping away. Was her brain intact? What to do? It was my call. She was not responding. I told the head nurse it was time to stop. The nurse looked at me in horror and disbelief, pleading with me. "You have to do something. She is only 16 years old. You cannot just let her die." More efforts proved futile, and I pronounced her. It was over.

I went to the waiting room to pass on the news to her loved ones. Tears, wailing, tears, wailing. Shock and disbelief filled the room. The girl's mother was grief-stricken and begged me to tell her that it was not true. Later, the family told me that the girl had been taking oral contraceptives and was experiencing leg cramps.

As I walked away, I thought that I would move on with my life now that hers was over. Twenty years later, it is not so. This girl from Philadelphia, whom I had never met before in my life, stayed with me. Reminders have come and gone. Sometimes I wonder: If I had been a little wiser and a little older, if I had tried harder, would she still have died? Would another 30 minutes of trying have saved her life? Now, at times, I am filled with a mixture of sadness, regret, guilt, powerlessness, and mystery. Why did this happen? Why can't I let her go? Why? Maybe there are just too many reminders. Maybe there are some experiences that you just cannot, and maybe should not, bury.

Seeking Forgiveness

MICHAEL A. LACOMBE, MD

If there is a common theme running through the submissions to the "On Being a Doctor" section of *Annals of Internal Medicine*, it is the story of the physician suddenly confronted by his own humanity. In form, this most commonly centers upon a dying patient, the physician overwhelmed by emotion, all at once aware of the depth of his or her caring. Much of the poetry submitted to the "Ad Libitum" section takes this form as well, such that together, we, the editorial staff, have come to refer to these submissions collectively as the "death-and-dying" pieces.

Far less common, but still submitted often enough to deserve their own niche, are the pieces we have termed the "seeking-absolution" stories, to which belongs the excellent essay by Dr. Costigan contained herein (page 102). These pieces, all having the sharp sense of nonfiction, center on the bad result. A diagnosis is presumably missed. A patient, through a presumed lapse, does poorly. The patient dies despite all measures. The physician-author, usually young and new to the profession, feels deeply responsible. And profoundly guilty. And unforgiven.

Why is this so? The answers, I have come to learn, are not so easily arrived at. (It has taken me some 4 months to compose this essay.)

The reasons for this recrimination are found in layers, the peeling away of which tells much about us, and about our profession. At the most superficial layer, but nevertheless no mean consideration, is the awesome responsibility that we are made to feel upon entering medicine—that, tinged with a secret sense of utter inadequacy. (It requires supreme arrogance for a young physician to feel adequately prepared for anything.) There is, you see, this crafty pedagogical trick we play upon our young trainees, whom we cause to believe they fight alone at the front, while all the time we roam behind the lines, supervising them in surreptitious ways. When a patient dies, the physician feels suddenly alone and the "tyranny of the shoulds" boils in the young physician's brain.

In my first month of internship, I had, while performing a thoracentesis, given the patient a tension pneumothorax. During the ensuing maelstrom of activity—with its chest tubes and intubation and older, wiser housestaff barking orders—I slunk away, caught in my incompetence, intending to walk away from it all, ready to quit the whole charade. The attending on the service, having once been there himself, caught me halfway down the hall, steered me into a side room, and talked me down off the ledge. (It was his example, I am certain, that would later render me sensitive to younger colleagues in a similar fix.)

At the second layer, and right under the surface really, is this sense of omnipotence with which we face the world, this imagined power borne out of the confidence we need, a confidence our teachers hope they have given us. We believe, especially when we are young, that we can do anything. When the inevitable death intervenes, we, too young yet to possess a "life view," feel to blame. The litany of tests, procedures, consultants, and therapeutics we might have employed suddenly becomes apparent. We could have done more. We are capable of anything, after all.

At a deeper layer, and related to this sense of omnipotence, is our posture of immunity. Young physicians are less careful about needle sticks, about communicable disease, about personal safety. Disease and death do not happen to them. Nor do feelings. Nor does the need to talk about them. Nor does the desire for a caring, sensitive ear from a colleague. Even if someone were to offer a bit of consolation, which sometimes happens, the young physician is not willing to hear it. (Older physicians are often as reluctant.) We shouldn't need it. We should be strong. We've been taught never to become emotionally involved. This was a lapse. It won't happen again. Next case.

But what is it that operates when you are seasoned and experienced in medicine, when you have thoughtful, sensitive colleagues to talk to, to absolve you—and, still, it hits you? Still, the guilt and recrimination boil up and overwhelm you. Where does that come from?

I had a patient once who traveled even more than I did—which was a considerable amount, let me tell you. George sold fire trucks to volunteer fire departments, and his job took him to small towns all over the United States. Six trucks a year was a good year. We would often meet in the waiting area at O'Hare Airport in Chicago to board the flight back to Maine. We would meet so often in this way that we came to look for each other. It became an anticipated part of the trip. We'd trade and switch and sit together on the ride home, and I could hear about central Nebraskans and rural Iowans, collecting characters for stories, reveling in the richness of it all.

And then while I was away on a trip and George was not, he became desperately ill and died. There was nothing I could have done, my partner said. But I couldn't accept that. Twenty years into practice and still I felt culpable. Had I been there I could have saved him. I was the only one who knew him. Only I really knew his case. Had I been home it would have been different. I should have seen it coming. That sort of thing. The guilt was oppressive. And there was no one who could ever understand.

Even now, years later, if I find myself at O'Hare, I look for George, forgetting for a moment that he is gone. Even now, it's still painful, so much so that I prefer to connect in Pittsburgh these days. It's that bad. As you know it can be. What I have come to learn—the root of what has bothered me about George—is that I liked him. And miss him very much.

But there is more here to this issue than caring for patients, although that is certainly profound enough, and the source of much agony for caring physicians. Why is the loss of the patient always so difficult, even when the patient is a relative stranger to the physician? Certainly knowing a patient well adds another dimension to the problem, but what is it that troubles the Dr. Costigans of the world?

A scene fixed in my mind sums it up, I think. Not too long ago, there was a house fire a mile down our country road. Driving by, I saw a dozen people sitting on a stone wall, facing a gutted home. Fire trucks literally surrounded the house. Hoses snaked everywhere across the lawn, crisscrossed even on top of a child's wagon in the yard. Christmas lights winked on and off from a nearby spruce. The front of the house had been reduced to a yawning, blackened cavity. It was a total loss. Those on the stone wall were the men and women of the volunteer fire department, and they had been fighting that fire most of the night. One of them, a young woman, blonde hair streaked with soot, had her arm around the shoulders of her partner. He was weeping. It wasn't exhaustion I read in their faces. It was despair—despair born out of the conviction that they could have done more. They should have been able to contain it, might have saved something, if only. It was a despair depicted at the end of the movie *Schindler's List*, when Oskar Schindler berates himself for not having sold his car to save five more Jews. It was the despair felt so commonly by rescue workers who arrive minutes too late, the despair lived by the emergency medical technicians, the cops, the social workers, the volunteers, who feel they might have done more.

It is the despair born out of basic human decency. Out of that despair, the Dr. Costigans of the world may derive a large measure of pride.

On Being Doctor Mom

CHRISTINE LAINE, MD, MPH

In my 4 years as both academic physician and parent, I have learned the following: The day that the babysitter calls in sick is invariably the same day that your children are battling a gastrointestinal virus; that you have 20 patients on your outpatient schedule, 2 of whom will require hospitalization; and that 12 medical students expect you to precept a session on medical interviewing. It is also likely to be the day before your most recent grant application is due. If your spouse enjoys the same career as you, he or she is apt to be 400 miles away at a scientific meeting.

I use hyperbole to make a point, but the frequency of such confluences of events in the lives of academic physician parents may help to explain the findings that Carr and co-workers have recently reported. A growing body of research demonstrates that women ascend the ranks of academic medicine more slowly, to lower levels, and with smaller paychecks than their male colleagues. Carr and co-workers explored the possible reasons for these discrepancies and found slower career progress and less professional satisfaction for women with children than for men with children or faculty without children. Like much good research, this study generates more questions than it answers.

Are the problems greater for academic medical mothers than for those in other professions? All working parents perform a precarious juggling act, yet academic medicine's work ethic separates it from other demanding professions. People get sick without regard for business hours, weekends, and holidays. Businesses close on holidays; hospitals do not. Unrealistic as it may be, patients want their physicians available 24 hours a day, 7 days a week, 365 days a year. Even though "on call" pressures diminish greatly after training, the guilty feeling endures that we must run whenever patients, students, or research projects beckon. We worry that our colleagues will disparage us (and they sometimes do) when we cannot.

Are things any better for academic doctor dads? At first glance it seems so—The fathers in the study by Carr and colleagues advanced in academia "despite" their children. Unfortunately, the investigators collected no data on the study participants' spouses. Had they done so, they might have found that academic physician dads married to academic physician moms were less academically productive than those with wives who have less demanding careers or, better yet, wives who do not work outside of the home. Juggling family responsibilities is a fact of life in dual-physician families, and the juggling probably impedes both careers. Further, academic physician fathers probably raise more eyebrows than the mothers do when they must forgo professional activities for family ones. In medicine's legendary "days of the giants," a giant rarely left work early to pick up a sick child at day care.

Why should medical schools pay attention to the needs of women faculty? Women comprise an increasing proportion of the physician workforce and may actually take academic positions more frequently than their male colleagues. Women are more likely than men to work in areas of need such as primary care, to care for underserved populations, and to deliver appropriate preventive care. They are apt to view health and illness from a broad biopsychosocial, rather than a narrower biomedical, perspective. Women also spend more time on the essential, though often neglected, duty of academic medicine—teaching. Academic centers need female clinicians to attract the many patients who prefer female physicians, and an increasing number of established investigators are women. Female faculty play an important role in the fulfillment of academia's mission. Finally, as more male physicians have spouses who work, issues that have previously affected only academic physician mothers are rapidly becoming issues for all faculty parents, regardless of sex.

Is there a solution? While some envision monumental changes in societal attitudes toward women and family as the solution, most academic faculty parents look for more mundane solutions. As Carr suggests, academic physician parents would welcome efforts to keep meetings comfortably within the confines of a normal workday. They would also welcome more explicit attention on the part of academia to such issues as parental leave and child care. Few female physicians take more than 6 weeks off after the birth of a child, yet data suggest that longer leaves optimize the mother-infant bond. Most are reluctant to take more time off because doing so will burden colleagues. When academic physicians become new fathers, they commonly take off little more than the time it takes to coach the delivery. The structure of many departments is such that having even a single person out, whether because of new motherhood or illness or even the death of a family member, wreaks havoc. Mothers, fathers, and others would benefit if academic medicine built some flexibility, through more faculty or fewer expectations, into its departments.

Nothing creates greater angst for parents than finding nurturing child care for the times when they cannot be with their children. Academic physician parents would appreciate institutional support in helping to ensure that such care is available. Unfortunately, many academic institutions do not have close affiliations with child care establishments. Such affiliations or the maintenance of a current clearinghouse of child care programs in the area would be an important benefit that institutions could offer faculty. Academic centers with high-quality on-site child care programs might even hold a competitive edge in attracting young faculty. Institutions should create child care programs that, unlike conventional child care situations, would give faculty the flexibility to work early, late, and on weekends and holidays, when necessary. Academic medical centers might even consider developing innovative day care programs for children with minor acute illnesses that preclude their usual school or child care routines.

It is unreasonable to expect that faculty who take substantial breaks in their careers to raise children will advance as rapidly as their peers who do not. However, on most academic tracks, slowing down for any reason can lead to derailment. Faculty who opt for part-time work, job sharing, or extended family leaves might welcome different options for academic advancement, albeit at a slower rate, as alternatives to leaving academia altogether. Some institutions provide such options but offer scant evidence that they truly condone them, and faculty may avoid them for fear of risking their academic longevity.

Like previous investigations, this most recent study of women in academic medicine did not specifically inquire whether women physicians were, on balance, content with their choice to combine career and family. Working mothers commonly lament about a feeling of mediocre performance at both home and work but would be loath to give up either set of responsibilities. Most do not blame their institutions for these circumstances but see them as expected tradeoffs for their own life choices. Many women choose positions that will afford them the flexibility they need to attend to their families. However, few choose to have lower salaries or less administrative support than their male colleagues with similar professional responsibilities, and institutions must recognize and rectify such inequalities. At least one institution has demonstrated the preliminary success of a multifaceted intervention to foster women faculty and remove unjust sex-based inequalities.

I would be relieved if, rather than sex bias, the reason why more women are not breaking through the glass ceiling of academic medicine is because their children are hanging on the tails of their white coats. Most of us are happy to have them there, and academic medicine offers a level of professional fulfillment, financial stability, and geographic flexibility that is well worth the juggle. The experience of parenting probably nourishes our performance as teachers, scientists, and clinicians. Nonetheless, it is distressing that Carr and colleagues' 1998 study suggests, as did one published in 1968, an inverse relation between child rearing and academic success. Academic medical centers must develop ways to support their faculty's efforts to combine two of the noblest pursuits—doctoring and parenting.

The Magic White Coat

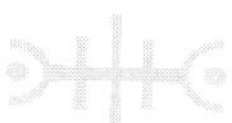

RICHARD G. DRUSS, MD

The wintry wind blows cold off the Hudson River at 168th and Broadway. Yet the medical students I see each morning at 8 o'clock, scurrying from one building to the next at Columbia-Presbyterian Medical Center, are without benefit of coat, hat, and gloves; they wear just their white coats. They are young and perhaps don't feel the weather so sharply. They might say that they can't be bothered by bulky clothes as they attend to their many patients. They might also say the tunnels that connect the disparate hospitals of the medical center add unrecoverable minutes to their already hectic schedules. But the young women and men seem to derive special warmth from their short white coats. Is it the grace of a uniform, like that of a freshly minted second-lieutenant, that fills them with such pride that they can brave the weather?

No, I think that it is the magic of the white coat. Given ceremoniously to them on matriculation, they must feel that the coat will protect them from much worse than the weather. (Forty years ago, in my day, there were always a few patients admitted for diagnostic workup or in lengthy recuperations from a stroke or coronary event—no longer.) Now, as they handle patients with resistant tuberculosis or AIDS, it must shield them from those deadly diseases. Perhaps even more important, how could these young people face so much human suffering—cries of pain, wasting away, the blood and deformity of disease—seen in any modern hospital, without their magic white coats as shields for their souls? It was only recently that they spent their days with the healthiest of people, college companions, among whom sickness (other than football injuries) was a rarity. Now every day is spent in the company of the very old and very vulnerable, who serve to erode their sense of youthful immortality.

They have probably seen death before: grandparents for sure, parents perhaps, and even friends. But not up close, day after day, in such quantity and such awfulness. And all of this is seen with eyes blurred by the fatigue of study and call. Never before have they felt so ignorant, so helpless, and so vulnerable themselves. They need something that will sharpen the distinctions between their patients and them. The patients are the fragile ones; they must be strong and vigorous.

So, as they rush along the cold streets from one building to another, from one patient to another, they appear impervious. Some may think that they are cloaked in denial. I prefer to think that they are cloaked in magic.

Death in Springtime

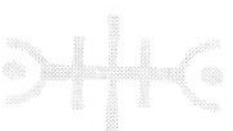

LAWRENCE SMITH, MD

An expression of shocked grief, a phone thrust into my hands, and the words falling on disbelieving ears: "She won't be at work tomorrow. She's dead." An accident had cut short the life of one of my interns. The story was tragic: last day of vacation, bags packed, a friend waiting at the hotel, and one final jog before a long flight home. A speeding car, a distracted runner, and an unfamiliar city combined to produce massive injuries, an ambulance rescue, intensive resuscitation, respirator support, and, ultimately, recognition of brain death. With her stunned parents at her bedside, the machines were stopped, and she left us.

She stood out among the housestaff. Her appearance was striking, yet she had an unassuming warmth and a palpable vitality. A hint of Europe flavored her speech, revealing her immigrant past and adding a touch of the exotic to her all-American looks. Always excited about working as a physician, she defined "joyful" for all of us. At the hospital, everyone liked her. Her success as a role model was never doubted by anyone who met her. No one was more alive and more incongruous with the idea of death.

As I hung up the phone, I knew that I needed to tell everyone about the tragedy. The bond created by the long hours of doctoring side by side makes housestaff a unique family; as the program director, I am the head of the family. They had to be told quickly. Whispered rumor was not the way to find out. Although I was nervous, I knew I would find the right way to do this. After all, I am a physician, experienced in breaking bad news.

We called an emergency housestaff meeting for 5:00 P.M. Find a room! Everyone had to be there, no exceptions. The chief residents did their job well, and as I sat on the conference table, the room quickly filled with tentative, concerned residents. What were they thinking as they waited and quietly talked among themselves? Did they think that they were in trouble? No. They sensed that this was about a tragedy. They knew. After all, they too are physicians.

When the room was full, I told them, "We are a close group. We all care about each other very much. Today is a painful, sad day for us. Klaudia died today in Madrid. It was a terrible accident. I'm sorry." There was shock and pain in the 100 eyes riveted to mine as each word brought home the tragic reality. And then there was silence, a long silence. Tears. Hugs. Caring for one another. Gradually, in small, tight groups, we left to find private places to think, to cry, to grieve, and to try to understand. It was so clear that calling the group together was the right thing to have done.

The housestaff came together as never before. Although they were already veterans of encounters with death, this was very different, so personal and so close. The psychological defenses that work so well in the clinical setting offered no protection from this devastating loss. The evening after Klaudia died, many residents were out walking the neighborhood streets until late at night. They were in pairs and in small groups, talking, grieving, and trying to make sense of this tragic loss. There were formal support sessions to help people deal with their feelings but, although these meetings helped, the greatest support came from the support of one another.

The memorial services, funeral, and burial were all rituals to help us accept the unacceptable. The pain and emptiness will lessen with the passage of time. Already a new group of interns has arrived. However, we will not forget that we lost Klaudia, one of our own, in springtime.

Brignole

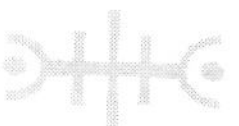

ANNE P. ROGAL, MD

I dreamt of Brignole last night. Once again I saw his handsome dark face and his slender form. He was dressed in khaki pants and the winter jacket my mother had bought him a year before he died. In the dream, we held each other in a long embrace.

His real name was Claude Louis, but as a resourceful young man trying to get out of Haiti, he had purchased a false passport and successfully completed his illegal immigration under the unusual name of Brignole Brisilien. Or was it Brisilien Brignole? Medical records never could figure it out, and I was never quite sure myself.

We met one night when I was an intern and he came through Emergency with headache and fever; the eventual diagnosis was cryptococcal meningitis. His grace and intelligence shone through from the start. I liked him, and it bothered me that after 2 days of receiving the correct antifungal agent, he seemed to be getting worse. Why wouldn't he even try to sit up or eat? He explained it to me simply: "Mon Bisket est tombé." He assured me that if it were replaced, he would regain his strength and he could handle anything, even that dreaded underlying diagnosis.

I went down to the cafeteria in search of James, the Haitian man who served behind the counter. "James, what's a Bisket? How does it fall down? How do you put it back?" He explained that a Bisket is a vertebra-like thing in the middle of the body. It can slip or fall out of place after a trauma, such as a physical blow or a fall. Replacing it involves deep abdominal massage using palm oil, "l'huile mascréti." You don't need to be a native healer to do this procedure, but you must have the oil.

The next afternoon, I met James in the cafeteria again. True to his word, he had procured the oil for me. This "huile mascréti" was dark and viscous, like engine oil, and emanated a musty, penetrating odor. I secreted the little jar and finished my rounds, then made my way to Brignole's room. I was grateful now for the hospital's outdated practice of putting patients suspected of having AIDS in private rooms.

"I've come to replace your Bisket," I announced. "I will do my best." I closed the door and silently prayed that neither maintenance nor food service nor nursing would find any reason to enter. Motivated by my own vague fear of AIDS, I put on a pair of gloves. Brignole was flat on his back. I coated my gloves with the heavy oil.

I had given a few backrubs in my day, but the abdominal approach was certainly not in my repertoire. Still, I had to do something. I placed my hands somewhere in the subumbilical area and, pressing deeply and slowly, began moving them in a circle. I didn't know where the Bisket was, what it was, or where it was supposed to go, but never mind. I pressed with slow, continuous strokes and moved a little higher.

It was remarkable that Brignole was able to relax his abdomen so completely. Normally I couldn't push so deeply on a patient's abdomen without eliciting protest. I continued, on and on, a little higher, a little higher. A wave of heat and dizziness passed through me. I was aware of the closed door, my physical effort, the strange odor from the oil, the intimacy of the contact, the silence.

"I'd better stop," I said.

"That's good," he answered. "Of course," he added, after the smallest moment, "it always takes three massages to replace the Bisket."

"Oh," I said. "Yes, of course. I'll be back tomorrow."

I returned the next day and followed the same ritual. Brignole was still not eating, still not getting up. I can't remember if his fever was gone or how his laboratory results looked. I knew that people need to have a will to live to get better, and I couldn't imagine recovery in his current state. I promised to come back for the third massage.

It was a marvel that nobody ever entered the room while I carried out these "treatments." What a reputation I might have gotten had the nurses discovered my activities. But the charmed privacy and the last of my precious oil held out through this final session.

I was pushing so hard that I seemed to touch the anterior surfaces of the real vertebrae. I pressed and manipulated this seemingly imaginary object higher. Brignole offered no resistance. Somewhere a few centimeters below the xiphoid, I knew I was done. At that precise spot, the Bisket seemed to have arrived home. I had a physical sense of completion. There was nothing more I could do. I left.

The next morning, I arrived in Brignole's room with nervous anticipation. Imagine my amazement and delight: The lights were on, the curtains were open, and Brignole was seated in the chair by the window, plowing through an enormous meal brought in by his girlfriend, Ysalie. He gained weight, improved, and left the hospital.

He and I never talked about his Bisket again, but we certainly talked about many other things. Within the structure of the doctor-patient relationship, we became good friends. Thanks to his own strengths and bolstered by zidovudine, Brignole remained healthy for nearly 3 years, except for some aggravating AIDS-related acne and one episode of sinusitis.

I got married at the same time that Ysalie, miraculously HIV-negative, left Brignole for another man. My husband and I purchased our first house just as Brignole was forced out of Ysalie's family home and into a subsidized apartment. I battled the National Health Service Corps for a fair placement, and he battled U.S. Immigration to enable his brothers to visit him here one last time. We both succeeded. Then he got sicker, and I became pregnant. I transferred his care to an AIDS specialty team when I went on maternity leave.

Abigail was born in December. Brignole died in February. Ungainly with postpartum weight, unstable in high heels after 9 months of supportive shoes, I teetered across wooden planks over the muddy cemetery ground to pay my last respects.

Of Locker Rooms and Labor Pains

ELIZA S. SHIN

Being a woman in medicine has its obstacles. I once expected that my gender would diminish in importance with each added year of schooling. That is, I thought that as my gray matter increased in prominence, the casing would become immaterial. As with many other childhood expectations, however, all that remains is a dream.

In grade school, cooties differentiated the sexes. Later, my secondary sex characteristics developed and remarks from the streets initiated me into the realm of womanhood. My intellectual awareness then followed, as college acquainted me with the academic nature of the feminist cause. These three—cooties, catcalls, and Virginia Woolf's "A Room of One's Own"—gave me a vague and distant sense of living in an unjust world. It wasn't until medical school that inequalities broadsided me personally. To heighten the shock, the first blow came from the institution itself, not from an individual person. School hadn't even officially started when a dean greeted us with these words:

"Congratulations, you are a class of firsts. You are the first class to use our new science facility, and you are the first class to reflect the general population. This class is composed of 51% females and 49% males.

Unfortunately, the brand new gross anatomy locker room was designed on the premise that the percentage of female students in medical school would never exceed 30%. So, the women will have to share lockers. Men, you'll have lockers to spare."

I had just agreed to pay my medical school $33,000 plus interest well into the 21st century and I couldn't even have my own locker. I didn't think much of this during the balmy days of September. As the days grew colder, however, my locker partner and I discovered that the feathers of three thousand geese would only be compressed into a 1′ x 2′ x 6′ space with the assistance of a battering ram. I'm sure the men next door wondered what that relentless pounding was as they frolicked about in their forest of lockers. Perhaps this pre-lab chaos was useful in that it prevented me from brooding over the task of human dissection. Thus, my soul may have been served. My problem-solving skills may have also been enhanced by the challenge of keeping my partner's street clothes free from bile stains and perineal juices. These elaborate rationalizations soon wore out my brain, and I was left feeling inconvenienced and out-of-place.

What architect drew up the building plans? Which professor gave feedback about the building's needs? Which board member approved those blueprints? I don't know any of those people, but I do know that none of them expected me. And they weren't expecting my daughters or my granddaughters either. That is, none of them hoped or dreamed that medicine would someday become a profession reflecting the general population.

Some women are overcome with self-pity. Others shake their fists at "the Establishment." Though I desperately try to wrench myself from the Victim–Valkyrie spectrum, I feel tempted to enact some form of retaliation when an attending calls me "doll" but my male counterpart "sir." Such "role models" ignore my achievements in the medical world and focus on my sex. Am I to follow their example, then, and focus on their manhood?

For example, a cardiologist led one of my physical diagnosis sessions. Outside the patient's room, he reiterated the seven-syllable physical findings we were to listen for, and, if graced by God, find. I entered the room, trying to remember the difference between Kentucky gallops and Tennessee horses, when my preceptor hailed the patient with a hearty "See, I told you I'd only bring you beautiful women." At first, I was stunned that an attending was capable of simple sentence structure. Then, after an awkward moment, I wondered whether curling my hair would have been a better way in which to prepare for this physical diagnosis session. As a wave of self-consciousness swept over me, I realized that my physique was being diagnosed.

After the cardiac examination, I began to notice other things. The attending physician I was to admire and emulate had disappeared. Instead, he had transformed into a tall and attractive vision of the doctor I hoped to be someday. As my thoughts wandered into frankly unprofessional territory, I berated myself and attempted to concentrate on his description of auscultative procedures of the heart. But hadn't those lips declared me beautiful? Was I not simply following the example of my attending?

Confusion and chaos reminiscent of the gross anatomy locker room filled my mind for the rest of my physical diagnosis session. Try as I might, I couldn't understand what was out of place. My attending's comment? His attractiveness? Me? If I left medical school, women would continue to be in the minority just as the architects, professors, and board members had planned. If I weren't in the locker room, we'd all be less inconvenienced. The attending could continue to view all females as objects of beauty instead of as future colleagues, and I wouldn't be frustrated by such distortions.

The frustration occasionally gives rise to the rage, which at times erupts at the drop of a hat. Once the fury is released, though, all that remains is rubble. What needs to be destroyed is not the species of men, but the ever-present fear that haunts women and reminds women of their sisters and their friends who have served as victims. Some men inspire this fear, and some men deny it. Unfortunately, the righteous rage often sours and, as a consequence, the Valkyrie makes all too many men pay for this fear.

Victim or Valkyrie. Is there another choice? Neither serves as a constructive option for me or for my male counterparts. In a feeble attempt to wax poetic, I searched through my mental thesaurus for words that begin with "V." Victor? Maybe in a few years. Vicious? That's for the Valkyrie. Valium? For the Victim. Venus? Hmmmm. A vision of the breathtaking Botticelli painting filled my eyes. There she stood, rising from the foam with the North Wind at her back. How exciting to witness the birth of a goddess. How enthralling to witness birth.

"Congratulations, you are the first class to reflect the general population. This class is composed of 51% females and 49% males."

If not for me, then 50%. If not for Lisa, Jane, and Ellen, then 47%. Each individual woman has made my class what it is: the first of my medical school's classes to reflect the population. Thus, in the 1995–1996 academic year, it will be commonplace to be a woman in the medical school community. When I grasp the magnitude of my position as a woman of the Class of 1996, I realize that I am on the crest of a wave that has been journeying to shore for years, decades, perhaps since the beginning of time. The despair of Victim and the rage of Valkyrie evaporate, and a sense of awe envelops me. A minuscule bubble of foam—myself—and 90 others unconsciously joined together to result in this birth.

This turn in the history of medicine, however, is not without its labor pains. Being called "doll" and being accused of sexual harassment are not pleasant experiences. Though the female medical students are the agents of change, the new heterogeneity of the medical community affects everyone. Old and young, men and women, patients and doctors, students and teachers must join together and nurture this birth. If not, it will indeed fail to thrive, and make victims of us all.

As I make my way into the medical establishment, I keep in mind all the girls behind me. They sit on the playground and play doctor while I roam about the hospitals and play pioneer. I hope that, by the time they mature, those girls will never feel as though there isn't a place for them in medicine. And maybe, by then, we'll have a new locker room.

The Privilege and the Pain

LINDA EMANUEL, MD, PHD

He stood at the lectern. He was in his 50s, a department chairman, talking to medical students at a quarterly pre-dinner lecture. He looked the part. As he listened to his introduction by the Master of Ceremonies, he held a book: He lifted it, then set it down, lifted it, then set it down.

He started his talk, a factual kind of narrative, easy to listen to. He was talking about the year he had served as a physician in Vietnam. He'd written a book.

He recalled the day he was called up, an intern at the time; he had phoned the 1-800 number to understand what it meant. Then he recalled the helicopters, the sandbag wall, the number codes—how many litter wounded, how many walking wounded, how many dead. He talked on, transporting us and himself into the reality. Sensations of receiving the torn and dismembered bodies of marines . . . boys. Boy after boy after boy. Day after night after day. He paused and lowered his gaze.

From the fires of hell he dropped us self-consciously back into our auditorium. Was he crying? He continued, but his thought sequence seemed to stutter. More pictures, sensations. Another pause. He adjusted his glasses; his voice hesitated . . . he recalled a 17-year-old with a triple amputation.

Take some questions. The audience rallied. Gentle buoying questions full of respect, care: awed students covering our collective pain as he had once covered ripped abdominal wounds with saline packs.

He works in shelters for homeless veterans in his free time—even now, our department chairman. Forty percent of homeless men are Vietnam veterans. Pause. Question. Recovery. He talked of coming home. No welcome, no room, no jobs for the veterans. Their agony under double lock—unknowable pain and vilification at home.

Pause, glistening brow, lowered eyes. Take another question. The hour is nearly done. He tells us of the boys who returned, who pleaded to go back to Vietnam, where the meaning of agony would not be shunned, shamed; where it would perhaps be blessed with death—who knows, maybe even with posthumous honor.

The applause was delayed, then thunderous. I went to the front and shook his hand hard, thanking him for his courage. He was strong, sweating, tearful, and gently smiling. "That was hard," he said. I asked to read his book. It was out of print; he held his last copy. He lent it to me, pressing past my hesitation.

The next week, in my outpatient office as usual, I saw one of my longstanding primary care patients; it was another episode of low-back pain. She too has suffered from post-traumatic stress disorder, from an entirely different experience, for more than a decade. She too has kept her life's structure together against overwhelming odds, being now a mid-level administrator. On my desk was the book I was returning. I told her of the lecture and my admiration for this man. We attended to her back and she left. It was many days later that I heard from her psychotherapist. He told me that my comments about this man had done something for my patient that I did not expect. I thought she'd simply be affirmed to know of this admirable person.

She was, but, much more than that, apparently she'd finally been given evidence that I was not afraid of her. I made him repeat that—I wasn't sure I'd understood. *Evidence that I was not afraid of her.* After so many years of care, could it be that I'd been afraid of her overwhelming pain? Could it be that this was so important to her?

A week or so later, a 42-year-old veteran was sent to our clinic by his shelter for a nonhealing foot ulcer. A 40 pack-year smoking history. Alcoholism. Multiple traumas. He was angry, didn't want to be examined. He barely stayed in the room. "Just my foot, not my leg," he yelled. Swollen; no pulse. I caught his gaze, apologized for irritating him, and explained why it was important for me to see his leg.

He flung off his pants. "Don't give me that," as I passed him a gown, "I ain't got no cooties. . . It's a dollar a peep." He sat down.

Amputation loomed and I thought of the boys in Vietnam. Had he been there? Yes. 1968. I told him about the lecture. Did he know the doctor who came to the shelter? No. But he was "glad someone sticks by us."

Did he have friends with amputations? Oh. His head flung back. "Yeah. Grown men crying." He showed me his 7-inch scar on his shaven head and told me how he'd been warned of death and how he'd gone out to drink himself to oblivion. No, he didn't die. Pause.

He tried a joke. Someone had asked him how he was today. "I feel like a dog." Since when? "Since I was a puppy." His voice cracked.

I finished the examination. No, he wouldn't come into the hospital or have an angiogram. Yes, he would take antibiotics and stay for arterial noninvasives. Yes, he'd come back. I shook his hand—hard. He apologized for yelling.

As he left, two nurses crowded around: "Who was he? We nearly called security." Just a boy with locked-in hurt grown old, I thought, surprised to realize that his threatening behavior had not registered with me.

I began to think of other people who let their pain show. I thought of times I'd felt great pain. I thought of how so many people seem repelled by pain. I recalled how our department chairman spoke, after his talk, of the silence and shunning he felt in our own medical institution, by physician colleagues no less. After years of seeing patients, I too had only just now been confronted with this startling fact: Pain is frightening.

Apparently, to heal, one must witness pain without fear. Pain pleading with weakness and pain masquerading as anger . . . no fear.

Had I been doing it all along? Not too well, I decided.

Eager to share this perspective, I told some sympathetic colleagues of this triad of experiences. One said it was a matter of seeing the critical meaning of an unknown experience, kind of like transcultural respect. Few of us have known pain, but we should be able to hear it and be respectful. Another said it was about transference and countertransference, about how we block meaning that we can't take. All people tend to be scared when we see pain. Yet another said it is like staying steadily with a dying patient, looking death in the eye.

But we all agreed on this: Healers can hear pain, healers give people permission to show pain, healers are not afraid to see pain.

Did anyone teach us that in medical school? Each of us gradually recalled a role model who had shown some kind of fearless healing. But we weren't too confident. I wondered if anyone really understands it.

Diagnosing at the Mall

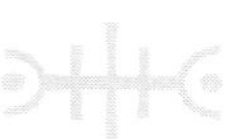

JAMES M. CERLETTY, MD

Physicians, nurses, and others who work in the medical profession love to make snap diagnoses. We pride ourselves on our clinical astuteness and the rapidity with which we arrive at the exact diagnosis of a disorder. A story was in circulation some years ago that illustrates this point. It seems that two clinicians were standing at a window on a lower floor of a Chicago skyscraper when a body, soon to be that of a suicide victim, plummeted by. With hardly a pause, one of the observers said "myxedema" and went on with his conversation.

Come on, admit it. You are making diagnoses at restaurants, at airports, literally everywhere. I can't tell you how many diagnoses I make when holiday shopping at the mall. I've made diagnoses in every area of medicine—from dermatology to neurology, from congenital defects to fulminating infections, from the trivial to the terminal. I have even postulated treatments that could be curative or palliative. I may share these diagnoses and possible therapies with my wife or another companion, but I never share them with the potential patient or victim.

This compulsive habit (or talent?) of making diagnoses is not unique to the medical community. Car mechanics on radio shows tell listeners that the noises in their cars are from the universal joint or a faulty baffle in the exhaust system. Grandmothers hundreds of miles away tell you in a letter what is wrong with your tomato plants. Music lovers tell the piano player which of the 88 keys is out of tune. Your mother-in-law regularly tells your spouse about your many flaws. But the medical community is different. We usually do not tell afflicted persons who are not our patients about their diagnoses.

My snap-diagnosis habit began in my freshman year of medical school, during the neuroanatomy course. Within weeks, my classmates and I were playing "What's my lesion?" We were doing the festinating gait of the Parkinsonian patient, the slap-footed walk of the tabetic patient, and the ataxic stroll of the patient with cerebellar disease. When I saw a cousin that summer, I thought he had syringomyelia, but it turned out that his peculiar gait was due to the fact that his underwear was too tight.

My physical diagnosis sessions in my sophomore year were taught at a VA hospital, so I thought that every big abdomen was full of ascites and that all pursed lips were those of smokers with emphysema. I was certain that the W.C. Fields look-alike with rhinophyma who worked at the corner grocery had a liver that went down to his knees and a chest wall covered with spider angiomata. As I entered my clinical years of medical school, my diagnostic vista expanded. I saw the Marfan syndrome at the mall, along with the more mundane varieties of arthritis, phlebitis, and episcleritis (versatility was my middle name). The little child in the stroller looked like a cretin to me, but I was sure his mother loved him nevertheless. In the public restroom, the man in the next stall seemed to be suffering from pronounced hypogonadism. Did I tell the victims of their maladies? Never!

As the years passed, the snap-diagnosis trait went from an obsession to a controllable hobby. I became blasé about obvious diagnoses. When my 14-year-old son, after passing an exophthalmic woman, said, "Dad, did you see that lady with Graves' disease?" I barely turned my head. I am now looking for the great cases. Woe to you if you ever become, in the minds of other physicians, a great case. A great case is, for example, a woman with supernumerary nipples and a different variety of cancer underlying each of them. A great case is a man with three testicles but no penis. It is someone with incurable cancer who now has an MI and a strangulated hernia. You get the picture. We medical people are obsessed with the grotesque.

My mall specialty is now, in essence, a search for acromegaly. This disorder, caused by the overproduction of growth hormone by the pituitary gland, leads to classic physical alterations that evolve so insidiously over the years that the patient and his or her family and friends are oblivious to the changes. The disorder is associated with enlargement of the hands and feet, prognathism, prominence of the brow, and a general coarsening of all facial features. Eventually, patients with this disorder all begin to look alike. The insidious nature of the evolution is characterized in the following example. Some years ago, one of the residents training in radiology at our medical center was a man with obvious acromegaly. I assumed that he had had previous therapy and that his pituitary tumor had been resected. On a day in early July, a new medical intern entered my office and informed me that this radiology resident had acromegaly. I answered that everybody knew that. "But does he know it?" queried the intern. When the issue was pursued, it became apparent that the resident didn't know about it ("You're full of ——," he said, when I suggested it). He had his surgery and lives happily ever after.

Since that July day, I have searched for persons with acromegaly. A few months later, I spotted one at an amusement park. While my sons were on the various rides, I made four passes at the man, clearly establishing the diagnosis in my mind. But I didn't tell him! I curse myself to this day for not stopping him. Perhaps he knew, but maybe he was like our radiologist, oblivious to the slow-growing tumor in his head. Since that day, I have steeled my resolve. I patrol the malls, looking for this disorder. Now I tell the patients about their suspected diagnosis. Don't mean to brag, but I've had some success in my acromegaly watch. I've had 3 previously treated cases, 2 new diagnoses (they took their business to another endocrinologist), 4 who couldn't be convinced that I wasn't an insurance salesman, and 6 who said "Beat it, Buster!"

Marrying Medicine

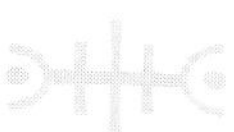

H.J. VAN PEENEN, MD

Dr. Mita Bannerjee inherited Miranda Amorelli on Friday morning. Miranda had been on a medical ward for 4 days. She was not responding to antibiotics. Nobody knew what was wrong, including Dr. Bannerjee, the new consultant in infectious diseases.

"I hate medicine," Dr. Bannerjee said to her husband that night.

"What's wrong, sweetie?"

She explained about Miranda Amorelli. But he couldn't understand the details. He wasn't a physician.

"Maybe I should just quit. Just be a housewife." But she knew she couldn't. Julian did not earn very much at Willamette's small private college. They depended on her earnings, or, rather, the promise of earnings to come. So far, overhead, uncompensated patients, and Medicare rejections had prevented her from collecting very much.

"Don't worry about it," Julian said. "You're not on for the weekend. Let the call guy take care of it."

That was easy for him to say. He wasn't responsible for Miranda Amorelli, who was one of those unlovable patients who seemed to be coming through the ER with more frequency these days. Miranda was a heroin addict. She was HIV positive. She had no useful veins. She was a noncompliant diabetic. She was belligerent and abusive.

She had no family. Nobody cared whether she lived or died.

So, Dr. Bannerjee asked herself, why should *she* care? Especially since she and Julian had the long weekend off and were treating themselves to an expensive mini-vacation, skiing over at Bend. She didn't even know this fat woman patient who had been thrust upon her. She wondered if the transfer to her service would have been so urgent had it been Monday instead of Friday.

Nevertheless, Dr. Bannerjee lay sleepless all night beside her husband, worrying about her new patient. Two hundred and ninety pounds, demanding, noncompliant, and foul-mouthed to boot. But sick. Very sick. And it couldn't be clinical AIDS. Not yet. There had not been the usual premonitory things, the candidiasis, diarrhea, feeling lousy. Just an explosive onset of severe infection. Miranda Amorelli had come in with a white count of 30,000 and a fever and despite 4 days on antibiotics was no better. As the Americans put it, she was "bad vibes." Finally, at 4:00 A.M., Dr. Bannerjee quietly got up and went to the phone in the kitchen.

At the hospital the night shift was winding down. Selma and Annette were standing at Miranda Amorelli's bedside where the patient was thrashing violently in what seemed to be delirium tremens. She had just pulled out the intravenous line placed with such difficulty on admission. She had punched the lab technician who had tried to draw blood and refused to have her blood pressure or temperature taken, striking out wildly whenever she was touched, however soothingly.

"She's Dr. Bannerjee's patient," Selma said. "We ought to call her."

"It's the weekend," Annette reminded her, "Dr. Bannerjee isn't on. Dr. Repscott is and you know what you'll get from him. Especially a combative patient he's never seen before. He'll just order a sedative and speed up her IV"

"He'll have to restart it then."

At that moment the telephone rang.

"Dr. Bannerjee must have a sixth sense," Annette said. "She's coming right over."

"Great. Let's talk her into putting in a central line."

Julian Benstetter, Mita Bannerjee's husband, was 20 years older than she and a sociologist who had met her while on a field trip in Kuala Lumpur. It was his third marriage and the first in which his wife was not a financial burden. Even now he had so much child support to pay that he was lucky to have found someone like Mita who could pay her own way and part of his. He was determined to be a good husband and never demand, never complain. Mita was already beginning to sound burnt out, so he knew he mustn't do anything to make her even more unhappy with her profession. But it wasn't easy to be a doctor's husband. He had sensed immediately when Mita left the bed and he knew why she had gone. It had happened before. Not terribly often, it was true, but more commonly than it should have and always, it seemed, on her afternoons off, when they usually scheduled their lovemaking. It was a good thing he wasn't young any more and could put up with that. Still, he resented it. Any patient, it seemed, meant more to a doctor than any husband. He was glad he was not a doctor himself, his mind constantly filled with someone else's problems. He wondered how young American physicians married to each other managed.

"It's all right," Dr. Bannerjee crooned. "It's all right. I'm here. I'm here. We're going to get you well. These ladies are going to help. You're going to be fine. You're going to be fine." She held Miranda Amorelli's huge paw in both of her own fine-fingered little hands. The paw was heavily bruised where one after another IV attempts had failed. Dr. Bannerjee had been crooning for half an hour and finally Miranda was beginning to quiet down.

"We need to get you well," she said finally, coming close to the patient's flushed and puffy ear, her voice gentle as though sharing secrets. "I'm going to start your IV, OK? You'll be a good girl. Hold still for me?"

Miranda responded by tearing her hand from Dr. Bannerjee's, grasping the bedrails, hauling herself erect and screaming. Lost in the scream were half-comprehensible words, most of them obscene.

"I won't! I won't! Let me go, let me go!"

"We can get some muscle in here," Selma said. "Security day shift's about to come on."

"A patient has a right to refuse any intervention," Annette recited primly. "It's in their Bill of Rights."

"She's delirious," Selma retorted. "She's not in her right mind. She can't make that kind of decision for herself."

Dr. Bannerjee sighed. These Americans with their odd preoccupation over non-essentials. "She is infected. She is dehydrated. She must have her IV."

"She'll just pull it out again," Selma pointed out.

"We'll do a subclavian."

The procedure was very difficult. Miranda Amorelli's obesity was such that it defied even the longest of needles, the thinnest of tubing. It had taken the IM Valium way too long to make her tractable, and Dr. Bannerjee knew that at home Julian would be getting up. He never said anything when she slipped away like this, but she knew how he felt. And they were supposed to be on their way to Bend by now.

She would give it up, she swore to herself. Stop practicing medicine, do her best to be the good wife she knew Julian deserved. But then she remembered her brother's contempt when she had left Kuala Lumpur with her new husband. "Just another woman," he had said. "All that education for nothing."

None of her family had accepted Julian. She had already shamed them by marrying a red-faced, goat-bearded foreigner after rejecting all the more suitable matches found for her. She would shame them more if she gave up her status as a doctor, status earned with such difficulty. What was more, she would shame herself.

Mita Bannerjee sat with Miranda Amorelli while 2 liters of saline ran quickly in. She watched the yellow bubbles in the catheter, checked the bag as it slowly filled, pumped the blood pressure cuff every 5 minutes. The nurses could have done that, of course, but they were busy now with morning report and there were other patients who were more tractable. And more attractive. Dr. Bannerjee could hardly blame them for taking Miranda Amorelli at her word and leaving her alone. Especially when they didn't really know what was wrong. Especially when she wasn't getting any better. Especially when there were no relatives around to make a fuss. Well, she didn't like Miranda Amorelli either, but it was her duty to care for her. She knew how guilty she would feel if, as the Americans put it, she "left any stone unturned." She decided to enrich the antibiotic mixture, put in additional coverage for anaerobes. Then her thoughts turned to Julian.

She was grateful to her husband. He had always been kind. Sometimes she wondered why he had sought her out, ignored the fact that she had already turned down so many men, almost forcibly taken her away, brought her here to the United States, improved her English, coached her through the difficult board exams. She hoped he loved her, but she could never be sure. He made much of giving up his career so she could have one. But she knew he had been denied tenure at the University before he went to Kuala Lumpur and that Lane College was probably the best he could do. Perhaps Julian had only married her because he knew how much money a doctor could make in America.

In any event, she was grateful. A woman should be married, even though she had been nauseated by her parents' choices for her, and although it was probably too late to have children. She was sorry about her family, now alienated from her, but she did not feel guilty about them, guilty the way she felt about this patient, Miranda Amorelli. For there was still something missing in her care. Miranda was failing fast. She must have *something* that could be treated. Bad-bug sepsis, pus under pressure?

"She's probably going to die," Mita muttered, half to herself.

"I know," Annette agreed as she made her last round of the shift.

And then it was 7:00 A.M. and Annette was not there any longer.

Mita shook herself awake. It was past eight o'clock. She had automatically curled into the high-backed convalescent's chair made for someone much larger and taken a doctor's catnap.

She called to the nurses.

"Give me a hand! It's time to turn her." The day crew hurried over to assist. They shifted the sedated bulk to its side. "Oh, my God!" said one of them, hand reflexively moving to lips. On Miranda Amorelli's backside the moist, black stench of gangrene assaulted eye and nose. Quickly, Mita pulled on gloves and probed the tissues around the evil patch. Fluctuance? She couldn't tell. The patient was too fat. But the superficial tissue was dead. And deep there must be something. An abscess almost certainly. With that white count, with the fever, with the uncontrolled diabetes, the thick, unresisting, relatively avascular fat, there could be any mix of organisms. It was obvious she would have to be drained and debrided. And quickly. "How soon can we get the OR?" she asked.

"There isn't a permit," the OR supervisor said. "We'll have to get a family member to sign."

"There isn't any family."

"Oh my! And it's an emergency? I'd better call administration."

More delays. Americans were obsessed with paperwork, so much of it unnecessary. Doctor Bannerjee and the surgeon waited with the newspaper in the Doctor's Lounge. She thought of calling her husband to explain, then decided against it. He would have to understand. And what could he say? If he said it didn't matter she wouldn't believe him for, of course, it did matter. The condo in Bend had been reserved for months. If he said it did matter and blew up at her, she would cry and feel guilty. He probably wouldn't blow up, of course. He wasn't violent like so many husbands, both at home and here, but he could project a silence. Oh, how well the Americans used silence! It would be just too terrible if her marriage should fail because of someone as intrinsically worthless as Miranda Amorelli.

"Uck!" The scrub tech could not restrain her disgust. The abscess was truly dreadful. The necrotic surface skin was undermined by foul-smelling cavities from which thin brown purulence poured.

"Kocher," the surgeon replied. He opened and debrided. There would be nothing left of this woman's buttock. Already the fascia was in sight. And anaerobes. Yes, certainly anaerobes. Behind her mask Mita began to grow angry. Why hadn't the ward picked this up before? Why hadn't she been called sooner? But then, how could one feel fluctuance in such a buttock, know what was the source of infection in so poorly controlled a diabetic? She couldn't blame the ward people. She would probably have temporized with antibiotics, too, if she had been the first one to see the patient. Still, she felt guilty about it. She shouldn't have waited this long before making the diagnosis. She should never have gone into infectious disease. She didn't have the temperament for it. Why not anesthesia where the hours were predictable and you didn't have to become involved? Well, she knew why. Infectious disease was the only fellowship available to her with her foreign credentials. So the personal demands of patient care were too much for her. That was just too bad.

Several hours later she finally returned home. Julian had long since made the bed and finished the funnies. She could see he was determined not to be unpleasant and sighed with relief.

"How did it go?" he asked.

"All right. She'll probably die anyway."

"But you did all you could?"

"Yes, I think so."

"Well, then," he said, giving her a hug as she slumped beside him on the sofa. "That's all that matters."

She kissed him gratefully. "I'm glad you think so," she whispered. "But it was an abscess. We should have known about it sooner. If . . ."

"Life is nothing but 'ifs,'" Julian said. She began to cry. Julian extended the hug and took her into his lap. He was not a big man but she was so much smaller he seemed huge. He was shelter, protection from the world, even from the demands of medicine.

"I'm sorry about the skiing," she murmured.

"Skiing's not all that important," he said. "And I'll bet your patient will live. You'll see. Did you get any breakfast?"

She shook her head.

"Waffles, then. It isn't morning, but what the hell."

She returned the hug. Why, she wondered, was he being so good? She hoped it was because he really loved her. But would he love her if she were to quit, if they had to live in near-poverty on his pitiful salary? She didn't know and she didn't dare ask.

Outpatient Clinic

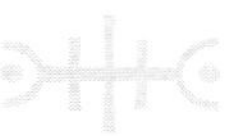

MITCHELL J. SCHWABER, MD

I think you'd better at least talk to her," the nurse said as she opened the door to my clinic office.

"Fine," I replied, "When I finish with the patient I'm seeing now."

It was Monday afternoon and I was in my weekly outpatient clinic. Every week patients come from around the city to my "cardiology" clinic. The fact that I am not a cardiologist but only a medical resident who sits next door to the cardiologist in clinic and consults with him when necessary does not seem to bother the patients, nor, for that matter, the primary care physicians who refer them to me. What is important to these patients and their doctors is the fact that I sit in a university hospital and as such have access to the top levels of academic medicine—including the cardiologist next door.

On this day, the clinic nurse came into my examining room while I was with a patient and said, "There's an old Russian lady outside who came to see you, but she doesn't have a chart here and didn't even bring a referral letter from her doctor. Even though there's someone with her to translate, I can't understand what she wants. I'm going to tell her to reschedule her appointment and come next time with a referral from her family physician."

"Fine," I said.

Since the doors to Jewish emigration from the former Soviet Union opened during the Gorbachev administration, more than 600,000 Jews have arrived in Israel. This emigration has changed the face of Israeli society, with Russian now heard almost everywhere. The health care picture has changed no less dramatically than the rest of society. In addition to an influx of Russian health care providers, there has come a whole population of patients in need of medical treatment. The Russian patients who fill our emergency departments and clinics are mostly elderly and often have stubborn diabetes, hypertension, ischemic heart disease, and the rest of the chronic maladies that affect the population of the Western world.

Caring for these patients has been a considerable challenge, not only because of their illnesses but also because of the language barrier, and, in some cases, because of a reliance on the part of the patients on their "old country" medications, despite the protestations of their doctors to switch to medicines used here.

Although I had not yet seen my prospective patient, I knew that just to interview her would be no small task, especially because she had come without a referring letter from her doctor. But no sooner had the nurse informed me that she would defer the appointment than she was back in the office telling me that I would at least have to talk to her. I surmised that the nurse's attempt to persuade the patient to reschedule had not gone well, and I realized that I would indeed be seeing this patient today. So I inhaled, looked at my watch, and said, "Fine," as I started to prepare my excuse for being late to my clinic across town later that afternoon.

When my patient entered, I had a hard time persuading her and her companion to sit down. They were both visibly upset. Her companion, an elderly gentleman who spoke broken Hebrew with a thick Russian accent, said he thought it was terrible that they had traveled all the way across town only to be turned away. I assured him that nobody was turning them away, and that his companion would be seen. Only then did they sit down.

My patient was an 85-year-old woman who walked slowly into the room, clutching a cane in one hand and her companion's arm in the other. He, it turns out, was not her husband or even a family member, but rather an elderly gentleman, himself an immigrant, who volunteered his time assisting other recent immigrants who needed help with translation. My patient had been in Israel a few years but spoke no Hebrew and had no family in the country.

I began my interview. The story was surprisingly simple. In front of me was a generally healthy but frail woman, whose medical history was significant only for hypertension that was medically controlled. She noted feeling a little "tired" when she climbed stairs or hills. The reason for her visit? About 6 months earlier she had begun to develop difficulty seeing because of bilateral cataracts. Her vision had deteriorated to the point where she could no longer read, and it was this disability that had led her to seek help. She showed me her appointment slip to the eye clinic for the following week. She was hoping they would offer her surgery. She had come to me because she wanted her heart examined before any eye surgery, to make sure it was fit for the operation, and also to get something that would give it a little boost of strength.

I examined my patient, looked at her electrocardiogram, and tried to persuade her that her heart needed no strengthening, and that I wished on all my patients, as well as on myself, a heart as strong as hers at 85 years of age. I started to write out notes to the eye clinic and to her family physician, and I noticed that all the tension that had been in the room when these two people had entered had vanished. Moreover, each began to express a gratitude that I felt was out of proportion to the service I had provided. As I talked to them, I began, I think, to understand why.

I also moved to this country not long ago. I remember, and still sometimes experience, the frustration, difficulty, and sadness of coming up against a system that is foreign and feeling that one does not have the means to master it. I thought of these people before me, two elderly people who changed countries late in life, for whom a visit across town was a whole afternoon's outing, who had to grapple daily with a foreign language and a foreign society, and who genuinely depended on the system to work for them. While even routine activities may become cumbersome ordeals for the elderly, the ordeal is compounded when one is in a foreign land.

I thought of my patient, whose only request was to recover her ability to read. And I thought of her companion, who dedicated his old age to helping others who had an even harder time than himself coping with their new lives. He assumed a role much greater than that of translator. He became her protector, the defender of her interests in a world that did not understand her. That she would be turned away from clinic, after having planned and traveled for so long, was an intolerable blow to her, and thus to him as well.

What dawned on me as I laughed in the office with this elderly pair was the fact that it was not just the medical service I supplied that made them so grateful. Yes, the news I gave was encouraging, but I sensed that there was more to their suddenly uplifted spirits than simply the relief that comes from a favorable medical examination. In their particular case, the mere fact that I was willing to see them validated the legitimacy of their concerns and their right to be there.

I began to feel ashamed that I would have been a party to their being turned away, and I was glad that the translator–protector had not been so easily deferred. I remembered the days after my immigration when all it took was a smile from a clerk at a government office to cheer me up, making me realize that there was a humanity on this side of the ocean as well. I wondered whether I had just become for these people the smiling government clerk. For a moment we had stopped being doctor–patient–patient advocate and had become simply three immigrants brought together in one room.

The elderly pair stood up. Each warmly took my hand and thanked me. I watched them as they left the room, on their way to the hospital exit and the bus: she clutching her cane and his arm, he walking slowly, carefully supporting her and guiding her way. I finished my charts in a hurry, for I still had to get across town to my next clinic. After about 10 minutes I left the hospital, into the

Jerusalem afternoon sun. As I looked down the hospital's front driveway I saw my two elderly compatriots, slowly but steadily making their way to the bus stop.

Balancing Family and Career: Advice from the Trenches

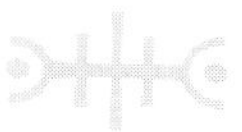

MOLLY CARNES, MD

I was recently asked to address a group of residents on the subject of balancing family and career. Although I had never considered myself an expert on this topic, I provided these young physicians—almost half of whom were women—with practical advice from my own experience over the past 14 years. Although many of my suggestions seemed self-evident to me, the residents' enthusiastic responses encouraged me to offer my suggestions to a wider audience.

Women currently make up a greater percentage of medical students, residents, fellows, and physicians in the United States than ever before. As a result, balancing family and career has become imperative for an increasing number of women physicians. This issue, however, receives little attention in traditional medical forums. Ideally, the art of balancing family and career is equally important to men and women, but as long as women are the traditional caregivers, this balance is more of an issue for them. This is particularly the case in academic medicine; because the academic clock and biological clock tick in synchrony, efforts to build a family and a career typically converge for a woman in her twenties and thirties.

Obviously, all families are different, as are everyone's needs and wants. What works for me might not work for others. Nevertheless, it is the prerogative of middle age to become reflective. In so doing, it has become clear to me that certain things have been helpful, even essential, in having a family and a productive career and enjoying both on a full-time basis. Although my own experience is as a woman in academic medicine, my advice may be useful to physicians of both sexes in other settings as well.

I am currently an associate professor in the Department of Medicine at a major academic institution. I was the first woman with children to receive tenure in this department. I am active in research, administration, education, and clinical care. I have two children, 14 and 10 years of age, and a partner of 22 years who is also a physician. I offer this information as evidence that my suggestions are drawn from experience and have resulted, at least to date, in successful outcomes.

To start, set personal and professional goals and plot a course toward achieving those goals. Look in the mirror and ask yourself, "Who am I, and what do I want to be? Do I want to be a department chairman? Do I want to have a national reputation? Do I want to be a parent? Do I want to work full- or part-time? Do I want to do research? Do I want to live in a rural or urban area?" and so on. There is no right or wrong answer to any of these questions; they are personal decisions. I periodically ask myself, "If something catastrophic happened to me today, would I have any overriding regrets about the way I have lived my life?" If you ask yourself this question and the answer is "yes," I encourage you to change something soon.

Once you have established your goals, be sure to choose a partner who shares these goals. Although I did not realize it at the time, this was the single most important decision enabling me to achieve both personal and professional success. During a recent conversation with several other women on the faculty, we surmised that women and men pursuing a career in academic medicine often view the ideal spouse differently. The average man in academic medicine is likely to seek a wife who will take care of everything on the home front—house, kids, shopping, laundry—so that he can spend long hours at work and feel nurtured at home. Women in this field, however, usually want a spouse who is willing to share responsibilities, negotiate tasks, and exist on a more equal professional footing. Thus, I would caution a woman to be wary of choosing a life partner who was raised to think that the worst form of humiliation was to be "beaten by a girl." I also advise women to avoid selecting partners who think that housework falls under the purview of the female sex. If a woman's goal is to be a tenured professor and her spouse's goal is to marry a domestic goddess, the relationship is doomed to fail. In my case, hiring someone to help with housework and laundry was the best thing for my marriage and my mood. For all the men reading this, I am here to tell you that dirty socks, underwear, and dishes are no more appealing to the x chromosome than to the y chromosome. The time you save is time you can spend with the kids, your spouse, or getting extra work done.

Strive for geographic proximity—that is, have all your activities close together. This is something I did not actively seek to do, but it turned out to be crucial in balancing everything, especially when the kids were small. I live close to work and can park right outside the building in which my laboratory, my office, and most of my clinical work are located. In addition, I have chosen to live in a moderately sized city where such things as day care, schools, grocery stores, and the pediatrician are readily accessible. In our city, there is a juggler who performs a trick in which, one at a time, he starts spinning 10 plates on tall sticks until all of them are spinning simultaneously. Once the plates are spinning, it takes only an occasional push to keep them going. If a plate is too far away for a push, it falls and shatters. The life of a woman or man with a full-time family and academic career is analogous to the spinning plates: Keeping all your activities spinning successfully is simpler when the distance between them is not too great.

To achieve balance among the various responsibilities of family and career, it is essential to have competent and trustworthy support people, such as secretaries, technicians, and child care providers, to whom you can delegate responsibility. You can then decide which tasks you wish to delegate and which ones you prefer to do yourself.

For example, at work I like to do much of my own word processing on grants and manuscripts, so I do not delegate this to the secretaries. I do, however, dictate all correspondence, memos, and less important documents. At home, I tuck the children in at night, read to them, and help them with their homework. My husband and I share such responsibilities, but I would not relinquish these joys to anyone else. In the same vein, you must always have a contingency plan. The school nurse will invariably call to tell you that your child has just vomited and has a temperature of 103°F when your spouse is out of town, your grant is due, you have eight patients in clinic, and you are out of Tylenol. I was able to enlist the help of an older woman who was always available on a moment's notice and, in the occasional crisis, could come to the house at 7:00 A.M. and stay until 6:00 P.M. You can work out your own system, but a back-up plan is essential for the well-being of your family and career.

You must establish priorities in your life. My husband and I make every attempt to attend our children's school performances or sports events and to ensure that we have some family time every weekend and almost every weeknight. I have never heard one of my terminally ill patients say they wished they had attended that meeting, served on that committee, or made that grant deadline. I have, however, heard many of them express regrets about the amount of time they spent with their children and family. After all, very few of us will be remembered for our professional accomplishments. It is far more likely that we will be remembered as someone's daughter, son, mother, spouse, or brother.

Get up 1 to 2 hours earlier than you have to each morning. My mother gave me this advice. She worked full-time, went to school, and ran the household. That extra time in the morning, when the house is quiet and your mind is fresh, allows you to complete tasks and arrive at work feeling like you have already accomplished something. Don't fritter this time away on routine items; use it to attack some significant project. In addition, use technology as much as possible to blend work and home life; have a computer at home so you can work while the kids are sleeping and a cellular phone so you can take calls in the car or grocery store.

While the demands of career and family may occasionally feel overwhelming, it is critical that you take care of yourself. If your health fails, it is a stress on the entire family. I look at myself as being in training all the time for the tasks I must accomplish as a mother, wife, physician, researcher, educator. As such, I try hard to eat right, exercise (but not enough to strain anything) and get almost enough sleep (at least enough not to get sick). Family vacations are also essential and can be very healing.

Maintain a sense of humor. I have observed that the most frustrating or irritating situations at work or home, when reframed, can also be the funniest.

One of the best aspects of "having it all" is having two potential spheres of support. Sometimes, at home, the kids or my husband are grouchy and whiny, and no one listens to anything I say. At these moments, it is heartening to go to work, where I get a little respect, I have some control over things, and I write orders and someone follows them. Sometimes things don't go well at work. Perhaps I get a nasty manuscript review, one of my patients is not doing well, or a colleague is driving me crazy. At these times, it is gratifying to go home and cuddle with the kids, bake cookies, read together, and be a mom. There are also those special times when it all comes together; things are going great at work and at home. These are peak moments to be savored.

I also derive satisfaction from feeling that I am serving as a role model for my children. My husband and I have shown them from an early age that the success and happiness of our family depends on working together as a team to accomplish tasks and solve problems. I am proud that my 14-year-old son has a very gender-neutral view of the world. I tell him that if he ever gets married his wife will really thank me. My 10-year-old daughter has no clue (yet) that her sex bestows her with any potential obstacles. When my children were younger, I limited my travel to one or two meetings per year, but now I am gone about seven times per year for two to three days at a time. These brief absences provide my children the opportunity to enhance their sense of independence. When I return, I discover that they are doing things for themselves that they were not doing when I left, such as making their own lunches and helping with additional chores. They enjoy bragging to me about their achievements. They also seem to have a renewed appreciation for me when I return, which I find very rewarding.

At this point in my life, I am enjoying some of the perks of a career in academic medicine that I believe can only be fully appreciated by a woman with a family. As you move up the career ladder, you are invited places to speak about your research or various other topics. When you accept these invitations, your hosts put you up at nice hotels with room service. Room service delivers a meal right to you; after you have eaten, you can simply put the dirty dishes outside the door. This is a truly delightful experience. In addition, in your own hotel room, you have complete control over the channel changer. This experience, it seems, is a novel one for many wives.

Another perk is the opportunity to be a mentor to others. I derive as much professional satisfaction from the accomplishments of former fellows and junior faculty members whom I have mentored as I do from my own. As one of the few tenured female faculty members in our department, I enjoy being in a position to give junior female faculty members advice that they simply cannot get from their male colleagues.

As with anything, there is a down side to "having it all." Balancing a full-time career in academic medicine and a family means that you serve many "bosses." The clinicians want you to see more patients, the educators want you to do more teaching and curriculum development, the researchers want you to write more grants and papers, and, of course, your children want you to be at their beck and call 24 hours a day. To prevent yourself from burning out by trying to please everyone, you need to set personal and professional limits. Decide what you want to do and what you are willing to do. Compromises and negotiations can be made, but try to emerge with your self-respect intact.

Another down side is meal preparation. When both parents work full time, it is impossible to provide a home-cooked dinner every night. If this is something valued by you or your spouse, my advice is to hire a cook. Our solution has been to have home-cooked meals on the weekends and, with good planning, as many as 3 nights per week. Thursdays are pizza, and Fridays are fast food. We all take a Flintstone vitamin daily. It works for us.

As women climb the academic ladder, there are fewer and fewer female colleagues or role models. I view myself as being just at the bottom side of the glass ceiling looking through, and, frankly, there are few persons on the other side whom I aspire to be like. This makes it a little lonely at times, and I get tired of sports discussions. Nevertheless, I am pleased to be guiding other female faculty members up the ladder and look forward to the day when one or two male colleagues will have to listen politely to an enthusiastic discussion of a sale at Marshall Field's.

Doctor's Orders

MARIA F. RODOWSKI, MD

"How can anyone possibly love me looking like this?" she asked me. She lay on her back, cradling the atrophic remains of her breasts. "I'm ugly. Why would my husband want to love me?"

"I think his love for you has to do with more than just your appearance. It probably has much more to do with all of the feelings and experiences you have shared."

"That's easy for you to say. You're still young and beautiful," she replied. "You just don't understand. He doesn't look at me the same way. He doesn't want me anymore. He doesn't want to make love to me. He's here only to take care of me. What do I have to give back to him? Once he was so proud of me, but now I'm a disgrace."

I couldn't argue. How could I, a third-year medical student, even begin to try and convince this woman, who was long past 70, that I had a better perspective on her marriage than she did? Although I doubted that her husband no longer loved her, I could certainly see how their relationship might have changed in the course of the past year as she struggled with metastatic rectal cancer. She had been raised in a society in which she was valued for her traditional feminine qualities; she was a good wife, perfect mother, and meticulous housekeeper. Now she was living day by day, changing bags filled with urine and soiling Depends with tarry stools. Gone from her existence was so much of her elegance, her self-respect, and her independence. Her relationship with her husband had to have changed.

Could I ask him to go to her and embrace her? Somehow this seemed far beyond my station. I tried to point out to her how he still did things for her, how he was kind and caring towards her. But this wasn't what she saw as missing. He was still there for her. He still told her that he loved her and always would. He had certainly not abandoned her, but she sensed that he was more of a caretaker than an equal companion. She would tell me how kind he was for putting up with her. She seemed to think that she deserved less. She drew all of her self-worth from giving; thus, it was difficult for her to receive.

"The chemo destroyed my body," she said to me when we were discussing whether she wanted to go through treatment again. "It made me so sick. The diarrhea was worse then. I was so weak, and I don't like wearing that pump around all of the time."

"If you do not want to go through chemo again, it's your right to decline. It is okay to refuse treatment. Only you know what you can take, and how long you can continue to fight. We are here to help you, whatever your choice may be. Don't agree to treatment just because someone is telling you it is the right choice. If it is not what you want, it is not going to help you to feel better. We don't guarantee that the treatment will improve anything—it's all a chance."

"Will I have to wear that pump again?" she asked, in a childlike manner.

"I don't know. You probably know more of the specifics than I do. Ask Dr. F. He can tell you the best approach. He needs to communicate with you, but you also need to ask him."

"He wants me to go through chemo. It is such a nuisance. I'm so filthy now, soiling myself like this. It is even worse with the chemo. I'm so tired of all of this."

"I want you to understand that you can choose to have chemo, or you can choose not to have chemo. It has to be what you want. If you are tired of fighting, that's okay."

"I'm not going to make it until next year. Why is everyone trying so hard? I'm such a burden to everyone."

"I think you are going to live to see next year. Perhaps I will not be here tomorrow, but probably I will. Perhaps you will not be here tomorrow, but it is likely that you will. I'm sure that you have made a difference in the lives of many people, and when you die you'll be remembered and appreciated. Isn't that what's important? It's hard to be sick and feel dependent, but no one is angry at you for needing help."

"Am I going to die? What's happening to me?"

I felt that I had exceeded my authority, but she needed me. I continued, not as a medical student, but as another human being.

"God decides when we die. I certainly don't know when. It is more important to enjoy what you have now and get the most out of the time you have. Please do that for me. I don't want to see you giving in just because you feel you should."

The Longest House Call

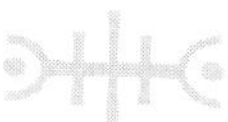

ARTHUR M. FOURNIER, MD

It took 1.5 hours to make the 700-mile trip from Miami, Florida, to Port-au-Prince, Haiti. The trip from Port-au-Prince to Les Cayes, approximately 110 miles on a paved road, took 4 hours. After spending the night in Les Cayes, we embarked in our four-wheel-drive vehicles on the 50-mile, 5-hour journey across the mountainous spine of Haiti's southern peninsula to the coastal village of Pestel. The next morning, a Haitian captain took us in a wooden sailboat to Anse St. Marceau, Au Basse, and Z'Etoit. These villages, just to the east of Pestel, are accessible only by boat. It took 50 hours to travel the almost 900 miles to Z'Etoit, our furthest destination.

We were visiting Haiti as part of Project Medishare. Miami, Florida, has strong ties to Haiti because of its well-established Haitian-American community. The University of Miami has several Haitian-American faculty members and students and a strong commitment to volunteerism and community service. After the embargo on Haiti was lifted, concerned physicians and nurses formed Project Medishare to provide medical equipment and supplies and to establish educational exchange programs to revive the health care system of the poorest country in the Western hemisphere.

In the mountains of Haiti, there are few distinct villages. The people live in homes constructed of thatched and woven palm fronds, spread throughout the countryside and connected by footpaths. Almost all of the children we passed on the road showed signs of malnutrition: red hair and swollen bellies. The Haitian health care workers who accompanied us assumed that all of the children were infected with worms. They had brought gallons of piperazine, which they distributed, followed by a handful of bread and a piece of candy, whenever we stopped.

Mere Maxime's house in Pestel started as a small home on the harbor. She expanded it through the years until it was the largest home in that coastal village. She insisted that we stay with her; staying at the village hotel, she said, would be unthinkable. The open-air porch on the second story served as both our dining room and dormitory. When we arrived, Mere Maxime, her daughters, and her sister prepared a meal of rice, peas, fresh fish, and plantains. They heated water in large kettles over charcoal fires so that we could bathe. Pestel has no running water, no sanitation, and electricity only 3 hours per night. Looking from the porch into the darkness down the coast, it was clear that 3 hours of electricity was a very local luxury.

The village of Anse St. Marceau (St. Mark's Cove) on Grande Cayemite Island stands on a dead coral reef no more than 5 feet above sea level. The houses, built of wood and plaster with palm-thatched roofs, formed straight rows: 3 to 5 houses deep, 20 to 25 houses long. Fishing is the principle means of subsistence—without refrigeration or transportation, nothing caught or grown can be shipped for profit. The people are industrious. Four large wooden sailboats were in various stages of construction when we visited.

We were visiting Anse St. Marceau and other locations on Haiti's southern peninsula to assess the suitability of these sites for rotations for our students and residents in family medicine. We did not arrive planning to make house calls; they just happened.

The first patient in the village who invited us into her home had daily fevers and drenching sweats. Her diaphoresis was so severe that a puddle actually formed beneath her on the dirt floor as we spoke. Miriam Frederick, the missionary–nurse who had involved us in this part of Haiti, made the correct diagnosis after asking only three questions in Creole. As we rounded the corner of the patient's house, we noticed a pit of stagnant water, dug for the animals. Mosquitoes leapt from it. In addition to giving the patient chloroquine, we recommended a layer of oil for the malaria pit. This was not good for the environment, but the pit was dug into solid rock, and there was neither a way to drain it nor dirt with which to fill it.

Once we started making house calls, we could not stop. It seemed as if every household invited us in to see someone seriously ill—a family with tuberculosis, an old man with arthritis, a child with cerebral palsy and seizures, a middle-aged man with a hernia. All conditions were diagnosed on the basis of directed history and physical examination. The pattern continued on Au Basse and Z'Etoit. On Z'Etoit, we saw an older woman who thought she had broken her arm after a fall. Her hand was swollen, but she had full range of motion of all her joints. We reassured her without the benefit of a radiograph.

Most of the patients we saw could be treated with medicines we had brought with us, with reassurance, or with the promise of future surgery. Our last patient, however, was different. She was on Z'Etoit, the most remote site we visited. Her family asked me in because they thought she was gravely ill. I found her sitting on the dirt floor of a two-room home that had no windows. Her family referred to her as a child, but her habitus indicated that she was a young woman. She was severely retarded, with microcephaly and withered lower extremities that suggested spina bifida.

Why had the family asked me to see her? It was clear that her problem had been present from birth. A brief discussion revealed the answer—the family hoped that I had magic powers with which to restore the patient to health. I could only praise them for the care they had given her for so many years and tell them "nou pa ka fé pi bon . . . courage."

There is no world record awarded for the longest house call. Even if there were, I doubt that ours would qualify; thousands of physicians have traveled further and served those in need for longer than we did. But this was a personal "longest house call." The journey home gave me ample time for reflection. Actually, the whole trip to Haiti was a "journey home" for me, in the sense that it returned me to the goal of "just being a doctor" that had originally motivated me to choose medicine as a profession. Haiti made me realize how much our career choices are dictated by our own needs—how much money do I want to earn, how many years of residency are needed, can I master the subject matter, will it stimulate me intellectually?—rather than by our patients' needs. The joy of helping people in such places as Haiti is unbounded by the constraints we face in the United States. No need to bill or collect; no "defensive medicine"; no technology overload; no demanding, hostile, over-utilizing patients; no petty rivalries between specialists and generalists. None of the statistics about Haiti that I had read in advance—lowest income in the Western hemisphere, highest infant mortality rate, life expectancy of 57 years, epidemic rates of tuberculosis and malaria—impressed on me the suffering of the Haitian people as much as that puddle of sweat on the dirt floor. My "house calls" in Haiti cost $400, for airfare, food, transportation, and lodging. Don't talk to me about cost-effectiveness. I'm going back to Haiti as often as I can.

"Ayiti te met yon hounga sou mwen."

Rise and Fall

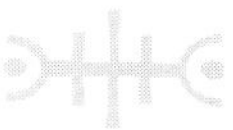

NICHOLAS H. FIEBACH, MD

I first met Dr. S when he was 87 years old. He had been referred to primary care by a urologist, who thought that someone Dr. S's age ought to have a general physician. I was immediately impressed by Dr. S's appearance. He was short but stood erect, deliberate in his movements, dressed impeccably in tweed sport coat and cap, and almost completely bald. He spoke slowly, with a slight accent. I tried not to stereotype him, but I could not help but be reminded of an old Zen master.

Dr. S was from Korea, where he had been a physician. He had gone to medical school in the United States and then returned to Korea. He eventually became the head of a large hospital in Seoul. When the Communists occupied Seoul during the Korean War, he was tried in a "people's court" and expelled from the hospital. He and his family fled the city and lived as refugees for several years. During that time, Dr. S organized medical services for other refugees. After the war, he returned to Seoul and directed the rehabilitation of his hospital, which had been plundered and damaged. When the restoration of the hospital was completed, Dr. S retired from medicine.

The elderly physician calmly told me of these events at our initial visit, with obvious pride in his accomplishments and resignation over the events that had disrupted his life and his career. He seemed upbeat and optimistic, however, as he continued his story. Dr. S had emigrated to the United States after his retirement and had become a naturalized citizen. His wife had died several years before we met, and he was living nearby with his daughter. He had two sons, one of whom was a physician in the U.S. military, and two other daughters, one in Korea and one in Japan.

I found a pulsatile mass in his abdomen that day. Ultrasonography showed an aortic aneurysm that measured just under 5 cm. During the next year, the mass grew another centimeter. What to do? The size of the aneurysm exceeded the cut-off for surgical intervention. Dr. S's general health was good. Was it prudent to perform a long and dangerous operation on a man almost 90 years old? The gerontologist with whom I consulted offered only that his approach was not to look for abdominal aneurysms in octogenarians in the first place. I gathered as much information as I could find on the risks of surgery and Dr. S's prospects if the operation was not done. Our best vascular surgeon recommended surgery, pointing out that he had done several successful aortic operations on 80-year-olds recently.

Dr. S and I discussed the data at great length, sometimes as patient and physician, sometimes as two physicians. I wrote him a long letter summarizing the information available in the medical literature. He talked to the vascular surgeon himself and discussed the surgery with his physician son. Despite all of this, he was not satisfied. Before he could decide what to do, he needed to know why this abnormality had arisen. He demanded respectfully to know the pathophysiology of his enlarging abdominal aorta. What was the actual defect, the specific cause of this problem? After all, he reminded me, he was not hypertensive and had no other risk factors or evidence of atherosclerotic disease. When I could only offer that the wall of his aorta may have weakened over time because of some inherited or acquired predisposition, he was disappointed. My attempts to convey Laplace's law and the likely progression of his aneurysm were no better because I was merely predicting the course of his problem and not explaining its origin. I grew frustrated as he calmly contemplated the time bomb within him.

A couple of years passed. He came for periodic office visits, always asking to review yet again what was known about aortic aneurysms. I came to believe that he had made a de facto decision not to have surgery. Then, one day, a call came from a different surgeon asking if I would visit Dr. S postoperatively. He had already had the surgery to repair his aneurysm and had sailed through without major problems. When I saw him later that day, he looked tired, but his eyes were clear, and he laughed despite his fresh incision. He had a slow but full recovery, and reached his 90th birthday as fit as the day that I had met him several years earlier.

During Dr. S's first visit to my office after the operation, I asked him why he had finally decided to have the operation. "Well," he said in his slow, deliberate way, "it was something that just had to be done." Then he laughed his typical laugh, and said nothing more. Perhaps if he could not understand the essential cause of the dangerous aberration inside him, the only thing to do was to eliminate it, whatever the risks or benefits. He struck me as more serene and indomitable than ever, having passed the tests of time and surgery.

Alas, his serenity and invincibility did not last long. He was increasingly beset by the vagaries of old age and minor but debilitating symptoms. His skin itched, he did not sleep well, his back hurt, he had trouble with his balance, and his bladder did not work properly. Now, with each visit to the office, Dr. S looked less like a Zen master and more like a failing old man. Although he still sported his tweed coat and cap, he needed a wheelchair to get from the street to the office, and he had to be lifted onto the examining table.

In the autumn, when Dr. S was 93 years of age, his daughter called in some distress. Dr. S had asked her to travel with him to Korea. She was sure that he could not make this journey, that he would end up sick and confused halfway around the world. His daughter was a senior citizen herself, and although she did not say it, I knew that she worried about her own health during such an adventure.

When he came to the office a few weeks later, we discussed the trip. He had decided to go to Korea so that he could visit the graves of his ancestors. I realized that the reasons Dr. S should not make the trip were the very reasons why he wanted to go. The telltale signs of his frailty meant that the end of his life was approaching, and he wanted to return one more time to the land of his birth and the graves of his ancestors. How could I tell him not to go?

Although too polite to say so, his daughter was angry that I had not forbidden the trip. Several months passed. I assumed that Dr. S and his daughter were still struggling over whether to go to Korea. When I saw his name on my appointment list one morning, I anticipated his visit with trepidation. I did not look forward to refereeing a family dispute or adjudicating his spiritual calling. Coming out of an examining room, I was astonished to see that the dapper gentleman walking steadily down the corridor was Dr. S. Dressed in his usual tweed coat and sporty cap, he was without wheelchair, without cane, without even the supporting arm of his daughter, who trailed behind with a smile. What had happened to restore him to health?

Dr. S had gone to Korea. He had prevailed upon his daughter, who reluctantly agreed to go with him. She said that he seemed to get stronger as their departure date approached, and the 18-hour flight passed without incident. He visited his family's ancestral gravesite and spent time with living relatives in Korea. Even better, he arranged to have a manuscript published by a Korean publisher. It recounted the patriotic exploits of an old friend, a man who had died without recognition because he had married an American. Now his friend's achievements would be recorded for posterity.

As his daughter narrated the travelogue, Dr. S beamed with satisfaction. He had saved the most remarkable part of the story to tell himself. In the midst of his journey to Korea, he had heard of the death of Kim Il Sung, the long-ruling North Korean dictator. The despot associated with the expulsion of Dr. S from his hospital and his home and with the division of his country had succumbed before him, almost literally in front of him.

Once again I glimpsed in Dr. S the same wisdom and equanimity I had felt the first time I met him and heard the story of his life. He seemed satisfied with his life but not ecstatic over the death of the

North Korean dictator. The Korean people were not clearly the better for it, he told me, what with the unpredictability and craziness of the dead dictator's son. And the death of Kim Il Sung could not change what had happened to Dr. S before. But the trip to Korea had clearly changed what was happening to Dr. S now. Whether it was the visit to his family's gravesite, the publication of his friend's story, the death of the Korean dictator, all of these factors, or something else, Dr. S was a changed and revitalized man. As he left the office that day, he told me that he had begun to work on his own memoirs.

Inevitably, the change in Dr. S was not permanent. The following year, various maladies recurred. Stomach pains began to trouble him and grew worse despite different foods and medicines. Eventually, he became weak and anemic, and gastric cancer was found. As always, he wanted to know all the details of his disease, to understand the pathophysiology. This time, however, he seemed more accepting of my explanations and readily agreed to palliative surgery. Several months later, he died at home at 95 years of age, still in the midst of writing his memoirs.

Atonement

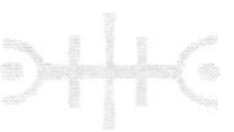

ORA PALTIEL, MDCM, MSc, FRCPC

I trained in a large university teaching hospital in Montreal. Our patient population was cosmopolitan. We learned how to interpret the silence of one ethnic group, the screams of another. The atmosphere was a tolerant one. Empathy abounded, yet patients had to adapt to us, come on time, wait their turn, and accept any piece of information or advice that we, with our white coats, had to offer. We supplied them with the facts, often without being asked. Although patient autonomy was respected, there was no question about who had the upper hand. Medicine and its practitioners were from the dominant culture.

Recently, things changed for me. I have become an immigrant physician, having moved to Israel 3 years ago. Knowing that I had come to an advanced medical system, I nevertheless felt that I had something to contribute. I brought my own brand of "good medicine" with me, hoping, of course, to do good.

A 70-year-old man came to my hematology clinic in September with a new diagnosis of lymphoma, only he didn't know that. Mr. D came armed with a discharge summary stating that he had had laparotomy for intra-abdominal adenopathy. The pathology report showed that he had diffuse large-cell lymphoma. I asked him what he knew of his diagnosis, and he answered that he had been told that he had an infection.

I searched his face for signs of dissimulation, disingenuousness. Mr. D did not seem to be the kind of man who would mislead himself or want others to mislead him. Nearby, his son sat and smiled knowingly. I took this as a sign that I might speak the truth. I did. I gently told Mr. D that he didn't have an infection, that it was a tumor, a tumor with a name: lymphoma. I explained to him that there is an effective treatment and that many people do well with this disease. I believed in what I was saying. I thought that he did, too. We talked some more. He was neither naive nor primitive. A 50-year veteran of Israel, he had worked in the university for several years. I assumed he understood. We made plans for further tests and for the start of treatment.

A week later, I received a phone call from Mr. D's family physician, an immigrant like myself but from Russia. He informed me that our patient was in a deep crisis, a broken man, pessimistic and refusing treatment. The physician asked me about the prognosis, and I replied in optimistic but realistic terms. He said he would try to convince the patient to return to the clinic.

Later, I heard that Mr. D had canceled his appointment for treatment. I asked the social worker to intervene. When she reached him, he told her that he was weak, that his fate was sealed, that there was no point. His son subsequently disclosed to her that I had been too blunt, too direct. Distressed by my miscalculation, I called Mr. D myself, asking him to reconsider. He repeated that he was too weak and would not tolerate any chemotherapy. I told him that we could tailor the treatment to him. I suggested that being a newcomer, perhaps I had not explained things clearly, and maybe he had misunderstood the message I had tried to convey. He agreed that this might have been the case. I wondered to myself whether the fact that others had not been truthful with him made him suspicious of me and my optimistic forecast. I invited him back to the clinic on Wednesday, just to talk. He said he would try. His tone was noncommittal.

I realized that this was not the first time my way of involving patients with their illness and treatment had backfired. My own set of ground rules ("Thou shalt not administer chemotherapy without informing the patient that he or she has cancer") was being questioned. I considered it honesty, an absolute value. Here, it was called being too direct. I had sometimes observed a conspiracy of silence between the physician and family. But I could see now that the patients might also collude. I had so deeply internalized "the patient's right to know" that I never even considered an equal and opposite right *not* to know.

I sat at my desk and considered euphemisms that I could have used. I understood that on the edge of the cultural gap on which I stood, I no longer had the upper hand. When I had moved to the Middle East 3 years earlier, I brought with me my household belongings, my children, my McGill University diplomas, and my Royal College qualifications. They all found their place. But I also brought my culture, my professional style. These had not yet found their place. All of the drugs and the doses were the same, but some of the norms were different. Friends of mine had worked in unusual places—with native Indians, in Africa. They were forced to adapt. So would I.

I recalled his imagery.

His fate was sealed.

Yom Kippur lay around the corner, and he believed it applied to him.

On Retirement

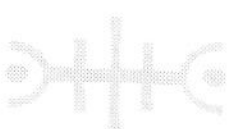

ROBERT H. MOSER, MD

Retirement is defined as "to withdraw from business or public life so as to live at leisure on one's income, savings or pension." This strikes me as terribly parched and resonating with doom, a dreary prescription for early demise. Yet there may be some truth in it. I am a veteran observer of unsuccessful retirements. I remember a tough, vigorous, 62-year-old four-star general who had commanded a corps in combat in Korea and an army in peacetime, each with distinction. I had the pleasure of conducting his physical examination for retirement. He had minimal stiffness and discomfort from mild osteoarthritis and moderate systolic hypertension but was otherwise in splendid physical condition. He could not wait to hang it up and devote his life to golf, hunting, fishing, and reading all the great books he had never had time for. Well, you know the story. After 6 months he was bored unto despair, and at 12 months was unrelentingly depressed. Within 2 years he was dead. The plot is all too familiar. And it is this plot that prompts me to offer a few simple insights that may be helpful, especially to young physicians early in their careers. Write them off as an old man's platitudes if you wish, but I believe that it is never premature to begin planning your retirement. And in these times especially, retirement may come sooner than you think.

Retirement is the final career for both you and your spouse. Make no mistake, if you have a partner, the two of you will retire together. No one retires alone. When your last graduate student has dropped off the family payroll; when you no longer leap out of bed at the crack of dawn in eager anticipation of defeating the freeway hassle and making early rounds before spending another challenging day in the office; when your trusted financial advisor smiles and gives you the green light; when you have sufficient assets safely squirreled away to enjoy the next 20 or 30 years in nearly the manner to which you have become accustomed; and, perhaps most importantly of all, when you and your partner really believe, after much discussion, that you will have fun living eyeball-to-eyeball, 24 hours a day, 7 days a week, together—in short, if all of these responses are positive, you are almost ready. But there is one additional requirement: You must have a plan.

This is your final career. And have no illusions, it is a career, and it will require every bit as much scheming and planning as any of your other careers. You may have some options after you retire, but they will be far more limited then than at any other time in your life.

Several prime ingredients make up a successful retirement. Some are a matter of luck and sound genes, but most are more controllable. Robust health is cardinal and most often represents a bit more than the blessing of genes and luck. At least 30 or 40 years of conscious attention to the controllables will pay off. I refer to such medical truths as rational dietary discipline, reasonable regular exercise, avoidance of cigarettes and excess alcohol, insightful management of stressors, and even using your seat belt and removing slippery throw rugs. You don't have to be obsessive about your health, just sensible about it.

It is tragic to arrive at the great moment of retirement in a state of physical disrepair, especially if it could have been prevented. How sad if, when you retire, you are no longer certain that you can handle the whitewater run down the Colorado River or tackle the Milford Trek on South Island—dreams you have been planning for 20 years or more. If you are in poor health, all of your physical options are severely limited.

Next in importance is financial security. You might assume that this should not be a problem for physicians; compared to most people, we are in excellent financial shape. Some of my wisest clinical colleagues, however, are incredibly naive about money. Brilliance at the bench and wisdom in the clinic do not transfer automatically to economics. These clinicians tend to underestimate what will be required in retirement to maintain their current standard of living. I cannot stress the importance of long-term association with a trusted financial advisor during your years of maximum earning.

The next facet of your retirement plan focuses on a realistic calculation of how to balance your intellectual, physical, cultural, and social activities. For each person and each couple, this balance will be different and very personal. Many long, serious hours of conversation with your spouse are critical to this facet of the plan. Friendly chats before the fire with good wine and soft music many years in advance of the final career may be the most crucial element in the preparation for retirement. You will be amazed at the infinite scenarios that evolve—shared dreams that may never have found expression in the rush of daily events.

I have many physician friends who seem incapable of having such conversations. They suffer from what I have called a "retirement lacuna." They love their work so much that it is beyond their comprehension to retire from medicine while they can still make a contribution. They will not discuss the subject. But there does come a time when one must step aside before it is too late. Some of the most pathetic figures in medicine I have known were great clinicians, true masters of the profession, who hung on too long. It is similar to the magnificent tenor whose voice has faltered or the champion boxer who has lost his agility. To compound the tragedy, none of the disciples of these clinicians can find the courage or heart to tell them to give it up.

When I encounter the physician who plans to die in harness, I become confused and sad for another reason. How narrow, how impoverished, are an intellect and soul that have not hungered to savor some of the intellectual, cultural, or social delights that swell beyond the world of medicine? Retirement does not mean that a fascination with medicine must cease. For most of us, this will never happen. But the pace can become slower and less demanding. We can read the literature with more reflection. We can be selective about the pro bono work we do. And retirement provides the opportunity to explore the vast, wonderful universe that the arduous pursuit of medicine virtually precluded. We gave our all to this demanding muse, and we did it with enthusiasm and delight. But now, at retirement, it is time to wander through those other untended gardens of interest that have been tantalizingly beyond our grasp. We have earned that privilege, after all.

Of all the elements in the balanced program of planning for retirement, intellectual activity is the most important. In my own teleological reasoning, I have always been taunted by the suspicion that some day, just as we have discovered endorphins and mysterious transmitters, some bright young researcher will identify other peptides that flow in response to intellectual stimulation. This researcher will find that they surge forth, bathing all organs in a felicitous, even rejuvenating, manner. If this is a fountain of youth, I think it springs from the higher intellectual centers of the brain in response to periodic stimulation. When this fountain ceases to flow, I believe that we see the mental and physical deterioration of the organism—I believe. This is my explanation for the phenomenon that all clinicians have observed for centuries: Without intellectual stimulation, the human organism withers and dies.

Admittedly, the best-laid plans do not assure success in retirement. Ill health is always an unpredictable villain. So is a serious, unplanned financial setback: "Janice just called from Oberlin. She's changed her mind. She doesn't want to teach Oriental philosophy next year after all. She wants to go to medical school! And Ted has decided to open a men's clothing store." Or, as you look up from your brochures describing the snorkeling off the Great Barrier Reef, your faithful spouse of 35 years looks you in the eye and says, "Now that you're home all the time, I think we need to give each other a little more space and free time."

But the ultimate catastrophe is to wake up each morning and just lie there, contemplating the day without the anticipation of joy. At that you must take aggressive evasive action to escape the demon boredom and its infamous handmaidens, melancholia and depression. This joyless awakening means you have made a mistake; your planning was badly flawed. You must step back and regroup to set the quartet in harmony once again, intellectually, culturally, socially, and physically.

Occasionally, a colleague will ask me whether I miss the action of being an active physician. It is a much more complex question than one might suspect. I have been privileged to savor several careers. But with each new adventure, one closes another door. This is never easy and is always done with regret. With every career change, I tried to maintain the connection with my other world. It never worked for long. The new job was so challenging, so all-consuming, that I was compelled to sever ties. I could not do justice to both jobs. I always had some lingering doubt about having done the right thing, but good fortune always smiled upon me. Each time it seemed I made the right decision and that it was time to move on.

Thus it is with retirement. There are occasional twinges. You never completely stop missing the sense of fulfillment that comes with teaching bright students, caring for the sick, writing editorials, helping guide the destiny of a great medical organization, or discussing global marketing strategies with eager MBAs. But you must fill your life with other fascinating things: those left undone or neglected, yet always within your peripheral vision.

Finally, let me discuss a most sensitive aspect of retirement frequently overlooked in other writings—the intimacy. My wife and I share a great deal. We love almost all of the same things, yet we are quite different people. Equal in intelligence, we have very different skills and interests. We respect this difference. We give each other space and time. It is an easy, unspoken thing. We argue, but rarely. And when we do, the one least invested in the subject yields, usually with good grace.

I wish I could say we divide the chores. We do not. My wife does much more than I. Yet I am beginning to *see* what needs to be done. A small point perhaps, but it has to do with fairness and keeping the peace.

Here is the sense of what retirement has meant to us, and a proposal for your own plan for retirement: You will enjoy the colors and scents of the flowers if you plan now for your final career.

The Knight of Faith

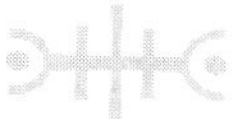

MATTHEW D.S. KLEIN, MD

> The Knights of the Infinite Resignation are easily recognized: their gait is gliding and assured. Those on the other hand who carry the jewel of Faith are likely to be delusive, because their outward appearance bears a striking resemblance to . . . Philistinism.
>
> Søren Kierkegaard, *Fear and Trembling*

A team of doctors was circled around a bed in the intensive care unit of the county hospital. The boy before them had just at that moment raised his head and disgorged a stream of blood into the air. It fell with a slap onto his white sheets and dripped off the side of the bed onto the floor. The bells on his monitors were clanging and the nurses were hustling about, offering him a basin and wiping up the blood on the floor.

Three doctors had pushed aside ventilators and ducked under thick, tense tubing to get close around the bed. Morning sun rushed through the windows, lighting the dust in the room and gracing the doctors' faces with an innocent flush. Old or young, they looked rich and strong in the Georgia morning light. They were listening to a medical student with a gray beard as he presented the bloody patient. A young woman at his side was his senior resident, a clumsy person with a degree in English poetry from Yale. And the handsome man at the foot of the bed was their attending staff, a well-published academic in the South.

The patient was a boy, and his face was heavenly white against the sheets. So unexpected was this sight at the county hospital, where the beds flanking him held two intoxicated and purpled men, that several doctors hurrying through the room paused and looked twice before moving on.

Just then the presentation was cut off when the boy gushed crimson onto his front. He paused to breathe, then jerked his neck a bit as a dribble of clot followed down his chin. He collapsed, panting. The attending swung left and right, then turned around, searching for a quick response.

"He's been doing this all night," said the medical student, tugging him back. "I mean to say he's been throwing up blood all night. The GI docs looked down in his belly, and they saw a . . ." he breathed, slowing the drawl, "they saw a stomach ulcer. He's been takin' aspirin, see, he's a wrestler. So anyhow, they saw an ulcer down there, it was bleeding, and they couldn't stop it, they said he needs surgery. You know, but with the Jehovah's Witness thing, we couldn't stabilize him for surgery."

"Huh," said the attending. "Are you a Jehovah's Witness, son?" He tugged at the boy's toe to rouse him.

"Yessir, that's right," the patient said.

"And so you don't take blood transfusions."

The boy coughed, turning his head to the pillow. A look of patience touched his brow, the look of those who are leaning heavily on recited facts.

"The soul is contained in our bodies. Jehovah has chosen my soul to see his face when he calls. That's when I die, I mean. Jehovah will not accept into heaven the body of one who is not chosen, and so I must keep other bodies separate from mine in every way. To receive them would mean eternal damnation." He had been groping on his bedside table and now produced a laminated card. "Here's a list of intravenous fluids I can't take. The saline you're giving me is okay. It's right there on the back, with a list of the okay stuff." With the recitation over, a look of fear and survival crept back into the corners of his face. Despite his illness, he was a solid boy, shining with youth. The medical student found a warm feeling rise when he looked on the boy, a nostalgic affection stirring the ashes of his own lost son.

The medical student was much older than his peers, older even than the attending staff. He had applied to medical school after his son died, in a twisting rage to escape the memory. In the hospital next to his son, he had once seen a burn victim who could lie only on bare nerves and so recoiled endlessly in bed. After Jason died, he came to know how that felt, and medical school offered an almost levitating escape. The physicians who had treated his son were above his laboring and punished kind. They confronted each other in clever Latin phrases that seemed to echo from ancient Rome. Their jokes were arcane. They seemed to never leave the hospital, to live endlessly and harmoniously together in a world of intellect and healing.

Now he was becoming a doctor himself, surprised by the cracks in that dream. But he knew that he was unique in his ability for medicine. He never told the other students about his dead son, always on his mind, but realized that he had been given a superior sympathy for the pain of the world. He had stayed up with this kid all night, just as he would have with his own boy. As the sun rose at 5:30, he had watched a few heavy raindrops falling off the trees onto the windows of the intensive care unit. The clouds were clearing from a storm the night before, and the sun was slanting across the brown city. At that moment, his heart had flooded with a vast and familiar pity for all things living. It seemed to him then that the pain of life was too great for humankind. It seemed to him that all people were bleeding like this at times, even those that appeared strong, that all people were hoping for resuscitation. And he yearned to help.

"The repair of your ulcer would be a simple matter," the attending was saying. "We could fix you in a snap of the fingers. But we need to give you some blood to do it." He stared at the patient.

"Ahemm. . . ." he throated, filling the silence. The boy was weak, but managed to grin in reply. The attending stiffened. "We're talking about you dying here, and I can't, I won't interrupt it if you won't take a blood transfusion. Ahem."

The team gaped at him.

"How old are you, my boy?" he said abruptly.

"Seventeen," said the patient. He was shivering.

The attending snapped to the bearded medical student. "Have you spoken with his parents about this situation?"

"Excuse me?"

"It's a simple question. The patient is seventeen. Have you spoken to his parents?"

The senior resident stepped in. "I handled that myself, sir," she said. "They're driving in from Macon right now, but I spoke to them by phone. The whole family has the same views. Jehovah's Witnesses. I explained to them that death is imminent without a blood transfusion." As if to punctuate this, the boy sprayed another cup of his own blood onto the cotton bed sheets. "They were very clear on the phone. They are prepared to let Jason die."

The medical student cringed. "There's more to the story than that," he said. "I called the county attorney this morning. She can get us a court order to give this kid blood. A court order, see? Then we can transfuse him. And she's waiting on our reply."

"There's no need for that," the senior resident interrupted. "As I've explained to our medical student, the decision here is clear. There really is no ethical way to justify giving this kid blood. He and his family value their religion more than the life we can offer them, right? We don't have to be paternalistic when patients are weighing their options rationally." The medical student heard the irritation in her voice. She kept her Ivy League accent from college and used it as a weapon here in the South. He knew she thought he was stupid, but she thought everyone was stupid. She was always quoting poetry to them, as though they were her personal tribe of savages.

"Can I have a drink of water?" the patient said. The student was startled at the transformation in the boy's face. Death was really nearby now, hovering around his dry lips and dimming the smile he tried to flash after speaking.

"I'll get some water," said the senior resident when the two men did nothing. She strode off to the sink and was back in a second, lifting a plastic cup to the boy's lips. She watched the water sink into his tongue, watched his Adam's apple tremble with the job of drinking. When he finished, he was exhausted and touched the senior resident's hand to push her away. She was startled by the cold palm that lay across her fingers, and her hands closed reflexively around his to warm them.

It softened her heart to feel those hands. The boy was so young. It wasn't that she wanted him to die, she thought. She wondered if she should be fighting for a transfusion, like the medical student. But she was so offended by the student's shallow impulses that she couldn't help opposing them. There were a hundred doctors like him at this hospital, pursuing a cure as if it were a spot on the map, swaggering out to rounds and drawling about their big saves the night before. Try telling them that disease was a subtle dealer, that each victory demanded a concession, and you lost them. Her attending was another good example. These so-called academics were the worst, all fighting to break into the literature that overwhelmed her desk. They were laughable and, on reflection, sad. Couldn't they see what a waste it was? There was too much writing. Even the very best stuff—Brenner, Braunwald—it, too, would be buried soon in mammoth volumes, indistinguishable from the rest. She missed her poetry, missed its humble fear of certainty, its parsimonious use of words.

"Give me the okay to call the county attorney," said the medical student to his staff. "Tell me we should give this kid blood. There's still time before his parents get here."

The senior resident met his eyes with disbelief.

"If I make the call now, we can have an answer in an hour," he continued. "He's bleeding to death, he's seventeen and he's gonna bleed to death, right here. We can still save this kid."

"His parents disagree," intoned the attending. He was wavering. "We can't overrule them."

"We can if we get a court order," he said, heading toward the phones. "What's happening here is plain crazy."

"Wait," said the senior resident. "Come back here." She lowered her voice to a harsh whisper. "What are you doing? Do you have any concept of this boy's basic human rights? No, wait. Have you even heard of ethics? You can't *do* this. It's his body. His decisions win, yours lose, every time. That's just how it works."

"But you're sending this kid to a death that doesn't need to happen. His parents are buying a world of pain that they're gonna regret. This is wrong."

His drawling confidence was too much for her. "Listen now," she said, as she tapped on the bed. "You might think you're Superman, here, stepping in and pulling life from the jaws of death. Well, get over it. Grow up. We don't save lives here anymore. We settle for a lower cholesterol or a higher urine output. That's what we do. And then they die."

"But this is not them," said the medical student. "We could save his life."

"Oh, I see. Here he is at last, the perfect patient." She gestured theatrically around the room. "Here he is, a boy who needs us to help him live! And he looks at all that medicine has to offer and he says 'no thanks.' He says that what we are doing is unnatural and ungodly. He preserves the purity of his body like a monk, and we bring him someone else's blood, we sell him something never meant for exchange. And he refuses! He suggests that doctors were wrong to dabble with God's ingredients in the first place. Infidel, you say! Well, I look around," she paused to let the ventilators rhythm fill their ears, "and I can't argue with him. Can you?"

"You bet I can." He stared her down. "And I'm pretty sure I'm right."

"Well, smarter people than you think you are wrong," she shot back. "Lord Byron, for one. 'Whom the Gods love die young,' he wrote. 'And many deaths do they escape by this; for the silent shore awaits at last even those who longest miss the old archer's shafts.' Listen to those words, will you? You save this kid today, the archer is still waiting for him, just a heart attack or a heartbreak away. He doesn't want it. Dammit, you're more scared of it than he is. He's ready to brave the archer right now, today. How can you tell him to wait?"

The patient was fading as she spoke, no longer really aware of the conversation. His eyes rolled back in his head every few seconds. The medical student felt he would burst. A familiar sense of loss was drowning him. He grasped the boy's shoulder, jostling it up and down. "You're wrong," he said, and the drawl cracked. "I know you're wrong because my own son was twelve when he took one of your 'arrows.' And I can tell you Lord Byron never had a little boy die of cancer, doctor. That's for damn sure." His eyes stung red but he persisted, turning his efforts to the attending. "If there was a way to save him I would have done it. My son should still be alive. This kid should live longer than today. You know I'm right."

The attending was provoked. "The parents have not given their assent," he repeated sternly. "This is all by the book. We can't give blood to someone who has refused it. We could get sued. We could be arrested for assault."

The medical student lifted his head to the ceiling. "You're right," he said. "We could get sued. We could even be arrested. We will probably have to pay for doing what is right." Then he turned to the senior resident. "You can't fight with medicine this way, you know," he said. "You'll go nuts. And you're too young. At the end of the day, you kick the questions out of the room and you try to believe. When it's quiet, you'll know. People need us. People need us to believe."

She looked at him, briefly speechless. The empty cup in her hand sounded a heartbeat click as she gripped it and released.

The boy had been trying to watch their mouths, but now his trembling became still. A smoothness settled across his brow. He lifted a hand to grope at the aging medical student. "Help me," he said. "I can't see. Why can't I see? Are my mom and dad coming? I'm scared. I'm really scared. Help me."

"I'll help you," said the medical student. "I will help you. He squeezed the boy's hand tightly. Then he stood.

"I'll make the call," he said. "You order the blood. Six units. O negative. There's still time."

Section II

On Being a Patient

Begin as though you were confronted with a problem: How can a writer make urinary incontinence delightfully funny and at the same time send a blistering message to that prima donna physician who "hasn't got time to pass wind" let alone have time for you? See Bauer's piece, *Star Treatment* (page 187).

What does literature have to tell us about the process of dying? Or, more precisely, what answers might a dying man find in the world's literature? Roger Bone, an icon of American medicine, wrote his *As I Was Dying* (page 262) during the last year of his life. It was published posthumously.

What does one say to, or do for, the disabled? Find out in Iezzoni's courageous and eloquent piece on page 277.

The "On Being a Patient" section of *Annals of Internal Medicine* publishes "short essays by physicians on their own experience of illness, accounts written by their patients, or accounts of the experiences of patients' families, with autobiographical writings on illness by published authors and fiction both welcome."

For pieces by physicians on their illnesses, see Waxman (page 210), Horn (page 207), Bernstein (page 214), and the overview by Spiro and Mandell, *When Doctors Get Sick* (page 201). For a wonderful portrayal in dramatic form of miscommunication between patient and doctor, don't miss Burns' *A Simple Procedure* (page 192). And for admirable expositions on the frustrating condition of being a patient at the mercy of doctors, read, as painful as it may be, Hansot's *Letter from a Patient's Daughter* (page 231) and Porter's *Venus on the Right* (page 254).

Patients are more often just in their criticisms of physicians than we are in our criticisms of them. They want to like us. They try even to love us. They make every attempt to accept our failings and move past them. They leave us reluctantly. They are quick to defend us, more so perhaps than we are of them.

Read this section and see if you agree.

Michael A. LaCombe

From the Green City

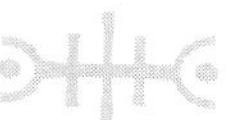

ANTOINETTE ROSE, MD

Willie wasn't really a hospital volunteer, but he liked to think he was. Not that it was so hard to become a hospital volunteer, but actually being one would have ruined it for him somehow. Besides, the application to become a volunteer—two pages of little boxes and lines—required a grip on reality that just didn't interest Willie. A few real things interested him. First, he liked the blue coats that the volunteers got to wear. Being resourceful, he managed a decent facsimile from an old work shirt that he found in a garbage bin at 24th and Kansas and just as soon forgot that he found that way. He believed, and told many people, that it had been his father's. He also liked the fancy name tags that the volunteers got to wear; those were beyond his resources but not his charm, for he talked a newfound friend in Personnel—bribed him with three dirty stories and half a pack of dirty cigarettes (scrounged from 24th and Utah)—into making him a shiny plastic name tag that just said, "Willie—Hospital Volunteer." He liked it that way, wouldn't have wanted or known or remembered what to offer as a last name.

Willie gave tours. He invented a history for the hospital to fill its past, invented himself and the patient people around him, invented them better than they could have themselves, and with more sympathy. He invented a leg for the man with phantom limb pain, stroked it with his fingers. He invented spiders on the walls for an old alcoholic, helped the old man brush them off his skin, steadied his trembling hands. He invented beauty in the homeless women, the women with no mirror to their name who still put on makeup, blotting their open sores, their louse and scabies scars, with thick indiscriminate pancake.

Willie invented health. It was what he did best. The patients took to seeking him out after they'd seen the doctor, just before they left, alone or in groups, by bus or on foot, to whatever their current squat happened to be. Some were strangers, hailing from the terraced lawns along Dolores Street or from the deep rhododendrons of the park. Most were locals, though, calling this or that heating vent on 23rd Street home. Willie's invention was always of use to them at this moment, to translate the doctors' words into something they could use. "He said rest my arm and I jus' got a job carryin' things . . . how can I do that with one arm, you tell me . . . ." "She said to ice it . . . how'm I s'pose to do that . . . don't even got a fridge!" "You think ice is hard, try heat in this weather!" "I'm s'pose to put these here eyedrops in, I got the shakes so bad can't pee anyhow but on the floor!" And Willie always had some wizardry to offer. He spun ice from cold iron; heat from the hoods of recently parked cars; steadiness from a sour-smelling, damp, moss-eaten wall, sending them on their way again, barefoot, homeless, and unchanged, but somehow refreshed, like scarecrows and lions and tin men back into the green city and into the fields of poppies beyond.

Star Treatment

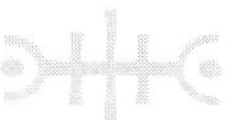

IRVIN S. BAUER

I wet my bed. That's how it all starts. "It was an accident," I tell myself. I am embarrassed. No more water before bed; maybe I was drinking too much beer. I am resolved. I am good. In the morning . . . the bed is wet. Peeing in the bed? Humiliation. Hide it from my wife. Put a towel down. Stay on my side. Don't turn. Give up sleep. Mention it to one of my pals, boyhood friend, like a brother, big-time CEO.

"Go to see my doctor. We've just given him a big grant. He's been anointed by a major magazine. He's just the best."

"I don't need the best. I don't deserve the best. I can't afford the best."

"Nonsense, nothing's more important than your health."

He calls. The earth moves. I have an appointment the next day at a major metropolitan hospital, famous for its care of celebrities. The waiting room is packed. Patients in two treatment rooms with another patient in the office. This guy doesn't have time to pass wind. My instinct is to flee . . . but my friend made the call . . .

Finally in his office. I am charming. He'll see I'm special. He'll want to take care of me. He stares at my shoulder as I talk. Not a good sign. "I wet the bed." He looks past me, then speaks. He radiates confidence, experience, and enthusiastic energy.

"I haven't got time for this . . . but for a friend of . . . "

Instant diagnosis. My bladder is overflowing. My prostate must be enlarged. Assume the position. Invade my privates. We need some tests. Blood . . . urine . . . ultrasonography of my bladder. "Make an appointment with my secretary. We'll start with medication to see if we can reduce the size of the prostate. If it doesn't work, we may have to do a simple procedure." Bing bang, he's off to the next treatment room and I'm on the street with a prescription for terazosin hydrochloride, dates for a variety of tests, a bag attached to my leg, and a tube in my penis.

During the next weeks, a new regimen takes over my life. I take my medication religiously. I talk on the phone a lot, and I've learned a new dance of avoidance. My wife, my plastic bag, and me. In the always clogged doctor's office, I have become "what's his name" at my weekly morning visit. The bag is removed. Zip, zap, in and out. I go home and wait to see if I can pee by myself. "Come back at 3 o'clock if it doesn't work."

I drink water like it's going out of style. I walk the living room. Lie on the bed. Stare at the ceiling. I hover over the toilet bowl . . . praying. Nothing. I rush back to the hospital. The tube is reinserted. This is done by a young associate. The doctor is off lecturing in Paris . . . at a symposium in Berlin . . . or has a special assignment on the dark side of the moon. I'm assured that insertion of the tube is a purely mechanical process and that the physician is fully informed of my progress. And so it goes for 6 disappointing weeks.

By the time I reach the elevator on my last visit, I am in agony. Every step is excruciating. I go back to the young associate . . . once again . . . wait my turn. Finally, he, smiling, adjusts my apparatus. The bill comes in later. Two visits—$260. This is no fun. The following week . . . quick visit, drop off a specimen. Physician runs by: "How are you?" Waves. Billed $130. I notice that the nurses in his office mirror his attitude . . . arrogant . . . aloof . . . superior . . . after all, they are the attendants to a star. I am lucky. "Be happy he made time for you at all."

The medication doesn't work. I go in for the simple procedure, affectionately called a "rotor rooter." There I am, lying on my back, spread eagle, my feet sticking up into stirrups, tubes inserted, television monitor tuned to this scintillating spectacle. The star enters the operating theater, gloves and mask in place. The lights are fixed. There is a hush. He looks at the monitor . . . dramatically pauses.

"Oh, look, there's a stone in the bladder." A stone? They had enough photos of my bladder to start an exhibition.

"It was hiding." Where? In my armpit?

Undeterred, he does something or other. "It shouldn't be a total loss," he says. He stares at the overhead clock all the while and tells me he has to catch a plane for the Virgin Islands. Finished. That's it . . . and he's off. Over his shoulder, a parting shot: "Don't worry . . . If you get into trouble . . . I'll fly back."

Trouble . . . what trouble? I wasn't told about trouble. This was going to be a simple procedure. We do it all the time.

I need a day for my body to heal before the stone can be removed. I am lying in bed contemplating my fate when this new spiffy doctor comes in to see me. One of the blood tests showed that I was a bit anemic, and my star had left an order for me to be seen by a " blood man." He asks me a few questions—age, weight, easy stuff—thumps my chest, listens to my heart, then tells me about all the blood tests we are going to do when I visit him at his office. "If that doesn't show anything," he says, "there are tons of bone marrow tests we can try." He is there all of . . . maybe 3 minutes. Later, the bill comes for my "comprehensive examination"—$500. What's the difference what is charged, they tell me. The insurance company will pay. Insurance industry medical facilitators . . . that's what they seem to be. But I don't have any insurance.

After a day of rest, I am wheeled down to the operating room for a second go-around. The star's associate, an experienced physician who grumbles about having to take over the "problem," steps into the breech. He is concerned and efficient and blasts the stone. It was huge. They show me a test tube full of fragments.

The star comes back from his trip and calls to see how I am. "Every time I try to skip a procedure . . . take a short cut," he says, "it comes back to bite me on the ass." He had left out the cystoscopy, a procedure in which they look through a tube inserted in the penis to see what is going on inside. If he did this procedure, he would have seen the egg. Oh, poor guy. What about me? I am the one who needed another 3 days in the hospital, another spinal, another set of tests, and the procedure, unpleasant at best, to blast the "dinosaur egg." Not a word about my discomfort . . . about the effect on my body . . . about my anxiety. I won't even talk about the cost . . . yet.

A week later, I go in for a check-up. The stone had caused the blockage, and it had been removed. The biopsy shows no signs of cancer. Good news indeed. If all remained the same after 6 months, I'd come in once a year to watch it, and that was that. End of story.

Three weeks later, I start to bleed when I urinate. Not a few trickles—gushes, streams of my blood pouring out. I call the great man. I tell him I must come to the office immediately. "Immediately" takes a week and a half. I call the office. . . . "Urgent," I tell them, "I'm bleeding."

The physician says, " . . . "

"But . . . but . . . but."

"I'm sorry, the earliest I can possibly squeeze you in . . . "

"But . . . "

To no avail. I consider going to another physician or to an emergency room. Then I think of the explanations...they'll want to see records . . . and . . . do more tests to verify. Anyway, he is the one who had . . .

A week and a half later, after a 3.5-hour wait...we meet. He takes blood and urine samples. We'll find out why I was bleeding. He calls the next day, somewhat agitated. I had lost nearly a pint of blood. Really? He does more tests . . . more ultrasonography to see whether the dinosaur egg spawned offspring or whether some other internal calamity is causing my blood to flow. The test results all prove negative. A cystoscopy then. We didn't do it the first time. We'll do it now. So there I am, back spread eagle in the stirrups with more tubes in my penis.

After a quick 10 minutes, we—my wife and I—are in a little cubicle for consultation. It is the prostate. The one that was supposed to have been taken care of. It had grown back, it had regenerated, it had multiplied . . . it was there . . . rubbing against itself . . . causing the bleeding. The physician draws diagrams . . . curved mountains . . . who knows. He is going to prescribe something that will stop the bleeding. The good news is that it has been known to stop or at least inhibit the loss of hair. It may even cause hair to grow. Terrific. The bad news is that it might, on occasion, slow my orgasm. The flow won't be as strong, that's all. That seems fair . . . a few hairs for a weak ejaculation. I don't know whether I am supposed to laugh or cry. I am numb, and I am still bleeding. How long will I have to take this wonderful drug? For the rest of my life, the physician tells me.

So . . . I start to take finasteride. The bleeding stops . . . and my body changes. I can't feel it anymore. Nothing. Slow the ejaculations? What ejaculations? I feel as if I am detached from the lower part of my body. I call the physician. "I don't feel anything. I'm walking around in someone else's body."

"Oh," he says. "Stop taking the medication." Casual . . . calm . . . an answer for everything. The medicine I was going to take for the rest of my life is no longer important.

"What's going to replace it?" I ask.

"Nothing."

"That's it?"

"The bleeding has stopped. That's the important thing. Make an appointment in 3 months . . . We'll schedule another cystoscopy . . . do a biopsy . . . maybe do another rotor rooter. You'll be fine."

Then the bills come . . . and come . . . and come. I was originally told that I would have to pay for two hospital days, one procedure, and one physician: around $8000. Instead, four hospital days, two procedures, and all that they entailed will cost me more than $30,000. My fault . . . no insurance. That's what I get for being an independent. I should have listened to my mother and become a dentist.

But what bothers me, besides the money, is the attitude. The physicians, the nurses, and the hospital couldn't have cared less about me. Health was just a six-letter word left out of the bill. And the great man . . . ? He may be a star, but he's no longer cast in my life story.

A Simple Procedure: A Play in One Act

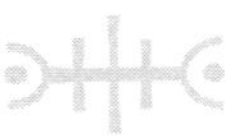

ROBERT BURNS, MD

Setting: A hospital room in a suburban teaching hospital. There is a chair to the right (stage right) of the bed with a large stuffed bear in it. There are a few books and a box of chocolates on the bedside stand. The door to the room is stage left.

Characters: Sarah Williams, 72 years of age. She is dressed in a blue gown and a matching robe.

Ken Porter, MD, 38 years of age. He is wearing a wrinkled white coat.

At Curtain Up, SARAH is lying in bed, watching the television that is located over the audience. KEN enters the stage after knocking; he does not wait for SARAH's permission. He is carrying SARAH's chart.

Sarah: Come in. Oh, you did.

Ken: Ms. Williams?

Sarah: Mrs. Williams. Sarah Williams.

Ken: Dr. Porter.

Sarah: Nice to meet you.

Ken: Dr. Janson asked me to see you.

Sarah: She did?

Ken: Yes, she wanted me to examine you.

Sarah: Well, she's already done that. Not to mention every medical student who's walked through those doors.

Ken: I am not a medical student.

Sarah: And all of the residents. I've lost count how many have been here in the past 3 days.

Ken: I am not a resident.

Sarah: You know, I may just start charging them to examine me. What would be a fair price?

Ken: What?

Sarah: A fair price? Let's say a quarter to feel my . . . This is my liver over here, isn't it?

Ken: Yes.

Sarah: Well, a quarter for the liver. And for my heart, it would be 50 cents. So they could listen to the murmur. That's what it's called, isn't it?

Ken: Yes.

Sarah: Then 50 cents for the heart.

Ken: I'm only interested in your liver.

Sarah: But if you want, I'll let you examine the liver and listen to the murmur for 50 cents. Think of it as paying for the heart and getting the liver free.

Ken: I'll just stick to the liver.

Sarah: You're a specialist, aren't you?

Ken: I'm a gastro . . . I specialize in the gastrointestinal tract. The esophagus, stomach. Bowels and the liver. I mostly focus on the liver.

Sarah: Just the liver? What about the rest of the body?

Ken: What about it?

Sarah: Don't you care about the rest of me? Wait, of course not. I gave you a great offer, heart and liver for 50 cents, and you turned it down. So, see, you don't care about the rest of me.

Ken: No, well, yes, I do. But Dr. Janson just asked my opinion about your liver.

Sarah: What about it?

Ken: She wants me to examine it.

Sarah: I already told you, she and everyone else in this hospital have examined it. Why you? Wait. Because that's what you specialize in. Right?

Ken: Yes.

Sarah: All right. You're the expert.

Ken: It will only take a moment.

KEN puts down the chart and moves toward the right side of the bed.

Sarah: What about the questions?

Ken: What questions?

Sarah: The liver questions.

Ken: Well, I've got them in here . . .

Sarah: In my chart?

Ken: Yes.

Sarah: But my liver examination is in there, too. Isn't it?

Ken: Yes.

Sarah: So you don't have to talk to me?

Ken: We're talking now.

Sarah: That's not what I mean. Don't you need to ask me questions about how I've been feeling lately or if I've been sick?

Ken: That's in the record.

Sarah: You said that. But since you're the specialist, I'd think you'd be able to ask me questions that the others didn't know they should ask.

Ken: Dr. Janson is very thorough.

Sarah: And that is why you don't need to ask any?

Ken: I ask questions if I don't see . . .

Sarah: For instance, no one has asked me if my bowel movements are blue.

Ken: They are? That's not in . . .

Sarah: I don't know what . . .

Ken: Are you having blue bowel movements?

Sarah: Is that important?

Ken: Yes! I didn't see that anywhere in here.

Sarah: So someone should have asked me?

Ken: Absolutely.

Sarah: But no one did.

Ken: I don't know how they could have missed something like that.

Sarah: Is it common?

Ken: Common? I've never heard of it before.

Sarah: Not even in books?

Ken: No. How long have they been blue?

Sarah: Never. They're normal.

Ken: Well, I . . .

Sarah: But see, no one asked me that question.

Ken: Ms. Williams, that's not something that normally happens. So they wouldn't routinely ask the question.

Sarah: Well, if I was normal, would I be sitting in a hospital bed?

Ken: No, I guess . . .

Sarah: So you know everything that happens to every person . . .

Ken: I didn't say . . .

Sarah: . . . and you don't have to ask me personal questions.

Ken: I have a pretty good idea about what happens with the human body and the liver when people get sick.

Sarah: Sit down.

Ken: I prefer to stand.

Sarah: If we're going to talk, I'd rather you sit.

Ken: I feel more comfortable . . .

Sarah: You want to be in charge, right?

Ken: That's not it.

Sarah: Yes, it is. Sit down. Move the bear out of that chair, please. My granddaughter sent it to me. Son number one lives in Seattle. That's from grandchild number three. Named after me, except she's called Sally. Move it. Put it on the floor, it's all right. A little dirt won't hurt it. (KEN moves the stuffed bear from the chair. He sits down.) Good. Chocolate?

Ken: No, I don't want any, thank you.

Sarah: They're good. Sunday school class sent them. Children? Do you have any children?

Ken: No. (Pause) I'm single.

Sarah: Oh. I saw your wedding ring. And I assumed . . .

Ken: I'm divorced.

Sarah: But the . . .

Ken: I just haven't stopped wearing it yet. Hoping maybe if I keep it on maybe I won't really be divorced. We're off the subject here. I need to examine you so I can get going.

Sarah: So that's it.

Ken: What?

Sarah: You just want to get going? This is all just a formality, isn't it?

Ken: That's not what I said.

Sarah: It's what you didn't say.

Ken: What's that supposed to mean?

Sarah: What do you think it means?

Ken: Are you a psychologist?

Sarah: Finally! A personal question! I thought you'd never ask.

Ken: Ms. Williams, if . . .

Sarah: Mrs. Williams.

Ken: Mrs. Williams, if you . . .

Sarah: Widowed, not divorced. Six years. I wear my ring for the same reason. And it doesn't get any easier with time.

Ken: Mrs. Williams. If you'd rather I not be involved in your case, then . . .

Sarah: What's a case?

Ken: You. Your care, I meant to say.

Sarah: Dr. Janson recommended you highly. (Pause) I'm not a psychologist. Bank teller. First National Trust. It was just First National when I started 43 ago; it merged a few years ago. I retired 4 months ago.

Ken: What do you think is wrong with you?

Sarah: What?

Ken: What do you think is wrong with you?

Sarah: What kind of question is that?

Ken: An honest one. I want to know . . .

Sarah: You're the doctor, a specialist, you're supposed to tell me.

Ken: But you must have a feeling, don't you?

Sarah: Everybody thinks they know what's wrong with them.

Ken: And what do you think is wrong with you?

Sarah: You know how it is. You always fear the worst or think it will be worse . . .

Ken: And what is that?

Sarah: You know how old ladies are. We get together once a week at the beauty shop and share aches and pains. After a while, everybody's sound the same.

Ken: So what is yours?

Sarah: Why does this matter?

Ken: I'm just asking a question.

Sarah: Since when do doctors ask a question like this?

Ken: So what's the worst thing it could be?

Sarah: Oh, you know.

Ken: What do you think it is?

Sarah: You're the doctor. You tell me.

Ken: I'm trying to see what you think . . .

Sarah: No one tells me anything. Just poking and prodding, one after another. All with a very pleasant smiles on their faces, or sometimes a dumb grin, and touching and pushing and pinching, and no one telling me anything about what is wrong with me. Even Dr. Janson hasn't told me what she thinks it is. And now you're here trying to get me to do your work for you!

Ken: That's not what I was trying to do.

Sarah: Well, first you walk in here and don't say anything, then you want me to tell you what's wrong with me.

Ken: I was just trying to . . .

Sarah: See how much the old lady knows?

Ken: Ms. Williams . . .

Sarah: Mrs. Williams!

Ken: Mrs. Williams. That is not why I did it.

Sarah: You know, you doctors are all alike. It's like talking to the wall over there. You don't listen. You just talk. And not to me. At me. Is that even talking?

Ken: I'm sorry if I got you upset.

KEN stands.

Sarah: You are not. You're just trying to get out of here.

Ken: You're right. I was. Just trying to bluff my way through it.

Sarah: Bluff?

Ken: I meant . . .

Sarah: You aren't really a doctor?

Ken: That wasn't the best word . . .

Sarah: Get out!

Ken: Ms. Williams, I need to . . .

Sarah: Get out! Now! Out!

Ken: I got started on the wrong foot. Then I tried something they tell you to use to help communicate with patients, and . . .

Sarah: They have to teach you how to talk to people?

Ken: Well, not talk to people but how to . . . Yes. How to communicate with patients.

Sarah: Didn't your Momma teach you that?

Ken: Yes. Well, not the way you're supposed to.

Sarah: And how is that?

Ken: Well, if you did the opposite of what I did today, you'd be close to getting it right. I'm sorry if I offended you. Doctor Janson can find another gastroenterologist for you.

KEN walks toward the door.

Sarah: Where are you going?

Ken: I think it's better if we end this relationship.

Sarah: We never started one.

Ken: You're right. That's my fault. And that's why I think it's probably best if you find someone else.

Sarah: You didn't answer me. Where are you going?

Ken: Out. Home. Probably stop and have a beer and try to make sense of what happened tonight.

Sarah: Do you always do that? (Pause) Drown your sorrows?

Ken: No, I don't.

Sarah: Walk away from problems?

Ken: I'm not walking away from my problems.

Sarah: You met a challenge, and rather than deal with it you're just going to walk away.

Ken: Mrs. Williams, I am . . .

Sarah: How come you can get it right now? When it doesn't matter?

Ken: Look, I'm trying to make up for what I didn't do right earlier. And if getting your name right helps, then it's the least I can do.

Sarah: Wasn't there an incentive before?

Ken: Look, this isn't gong to work for either of us. So I'm just going to leave, and—oh, never mind.

Sarah: Sit down.

Ken: What?

Sarah: You heard me. Sit down.

Ken: I'm leaving, and I don't want to . . .

Sarah: You're supposed to be the best. Prove it. Sit down right there; I don't want you standing. I want us to be at the same level. (KEN sits.) There.

Ken: Now what?

Sarah: Start

Ken: Start what? A fight?

Sarah: No, that's my part. Ask me your questions.

Ken: What questions?

Sarah: Are you really the best Dr. Janson can find? Your liver questions. Here, I'll get you started. I don't have blue bowel movements.

Ken: No, I can't, not this . . .

KEN stands and walks toward the door.

Sarah: Where are you going? I didn't say you could leave.

KEN leaves the room, re-enters, and walks toward the side of the bed.

Ken: Hello, Mrs. Williams. I'm Dr. Ken Porter. I'd like to ask you a few questions.

Sarah: (Pause) Please sit down.

KEN sits down in the chair.

Ken: Please, tell me a little about yourself.

Sarah: I haven't been feeling good for a while. And I'm afraid I have cancer.

(Lights fade.)

When Doctors Get Sick

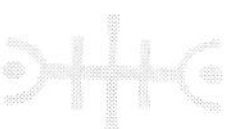

HOWARD M. SPIRO, MD
HARVEY N. MANDELL, MD

Storytelling has gained prominence in medicine, where the tales of the sick are medicalized as "pathography." Interest in "narrative," as it is called in academic circles, is equally widespread in history, where stories based on facts and re-created with imagination bring other times to life more dramatically than the dry data of economics and biography. If we physicians read more accounts of our patients' travails and, better still, talked about them with each other, we might improve the humane qualities of medical care. The chiaroscuro of conversation and narrative can so highlight the social, emotional, and economic origins of many complaints that it might even help to make medical practice more cost-effective.

We review here what the two of us learned from the stories about sick doctors that we collected a decade ago (*When Doctors Get Sick*, New York: Plenum, 1987). These narratives illuminate the dilemma of impaired physicians—or wounded healers, as they have been called—that our profession must examine before others do it for us.

Being seriously ill or disabled gives doctors a foretaste of retirement and the leisure for reveries that their duties have taken from them; it makes them contemplate even their own death. The stories of sick doctors force emotion back into medicine, and when sick doctors themselves learn the comfort that comes from attention and devotion, empathy cannot lag far behind. Practitioners of alternative medicine already know this, their popularity growing in part because they delight their patients with time and attention.

More than most people, sick doctors deny that they are sick. They may worry privately about their health, but the unconscious pact with the Creator that many physicians have made—we will take care of the sick and You will guarantee us good health—makes it hard for them to realize that they, too, are mortal. The hypochondriasis of medical school contributes to easy denial, because when physicians fear one disease after another and find them all phantom, they come to believe in their own invulnerability. Only unrelenting pain, great weight loss, or catastrophic bleeding confirmed by the evidence of radiography or endoscopy awaken them to the reality that they have become patients.

Trained detachment has been praised since Osler's time. "Don't get too involved," older doctors still advise. Their younger colleagues then rehearse equanimity and soon lose their emotions. Professional detachment spreads from office to home, turning into a kind of alexithymia so that many physicians no longer recognize when or if they have any emotion at all. Denial is further fostered by the silence of fellow physicians. In a hospital, the "No Visitors" sign on a doctor-patient's sickroom door may be put up not so much to spare him or her from too many guests as to permit colleagues still vertical to pass by without guilt.

When the delayed realization of illness dawns, long-practiced detachment leads to distance and isolation. Sick doctors often deny foreboding and boast of their composure as if emotion were shameful, because that is how we physicians want our patients to behave. We praise the noncomplainer who does not flinch at liver biopsy and the postoperative patient who jokes rather than moans.

There are other reasons why sick doctors try to be good patients who do what they are told without complaint. One may be that sick doctors hope to return to an active professional life. Admitting a need for emotional comfort might embarrass their attending physicians, which could make for uncomfortable professional relations later on.

When a doctor is sick, especially in a hospital, he or she undergoes a role reversal. Strangely, the doctor is the patient, and the familiar aspects of the hospital are unrecognizable from a stretcher. Loss of control is hardest of all for sick doctors, so used are they to the obedience of others: Sick radiologists try to read their own films, and the bed-bound physician strains to scan the bedside monitor. Sick doctors are lonely patients, isolated but on watch, vigilant against error. Caught in the double bind of wanting to be a good patient yet worrying about what can go wrong, most sick doctors watch their colleagues as closely as they fear their colleagues are watching them. It is not easy to be a doctor and a patient all at once.

The narratives of doctors who have heart attacks or angina show how exquisitely sensitive sick doctors have become to the reality of their own symptoms, even though they have been trained—even paid—to attend mainly to the findings of computed tomography or endoscopy. They learn the truth of what Elaine Scarry has written: "To have pain is to be certain: To hear about pain is to be in doubt."

Nor is it easy to be a doctor taking care of another doctor, for physicians often give doctor-patients credit for knowing more than they really do. They spare their doctor-patients the rituals that other patients must endure. Leaving out the rectal examination is bad enough, but even worse are the occasions when attending physicians are too delicate to inquire about personal problems. This causes doctor-patients to undergo many tests "for completeness" when a little conversation about life and stress might have brought out important issues and eliminated any need for diagnostic studies. If doctors have a personal physician at all, they are likely to have chosen a coeval, which lessens the likelihood of objectivity from the very start. As physicians age, they may be startled to realize that their doctor has grown older, also: A 75-year-old physician might find that he or she is getting care from another 75-year-old physician who is nearing retirement and practicing part-time.

Guilt worsens the plight of the doctor who falls sick. Traditionally, physicians have been such workaholics that they are anxious to continue regardless of risk to their patients. Because they often define themselves by their work, physicians work harder than ever to justify themselves when things are not going right. Some sick doctors claim that they work to meet expenses, but it seems more likely that an exaggerated sense of duty is responsible: Sick doctors often brag about how long they continued to practice despite growing disability. Yet praising seriously ill doctors for dragging themselves to the hospital to make rounds overlooks the harm that impaired physicians may do their patients.

Any patient's response to illness depends upon nature, character, and "premorbid" personality, upon age and accomplishment. Ten years ago, religion brought very little comfort to most doctor-patients, but that may be changing as spiritual matters gain more attention. Old people can grasp the horizon at last, and they fear death far less than the young. It is a prolonged and painful dying that worries us all.

The accounts of sick doctors raise doubts about some popular ethical concerns, such as autonomy, parentalism (formerly called "paternalism"), and truth-telling. Autonomy finds little favor with sick doctors, who are mostly relieved when another physician takes over their case. Sick doctors, in our experience at least, did not want too much detail; they trusted their physicians to be loyal to them. We doctors may represent a special kind of patient because we identify with each other, but medical practice has meant being loyal to our patients' interests at all times, even under managed care. A judicious parentalism may be in order: Many sick doctors have written about the peace of mind that comes when they no longer had to face one decision after another. After all, most sick patients have clouded judgment, as physicians used to know.

Although truth-telling has turned into a prime medical ethic, more important than empathy or kindness, hard truths are sometimes unwelcome to sick doctors, who yearn for compassion and kindness, faith and hope. Doctors should not begin to lie again to their patients—physicians or laity—but should understand how much hope, consolation, and optimism can help.

Doctors will continue to get sick and other doctors will treat them, and sick doctors, thanks to their medical training, will have unique problems and unique perplexities. What can be done to prepare for such problems? Of the many ideas that come to mind, a regular "checkup," like those doctors urge on their patients, seems foremost.

Early in their first year of medical school, students should undergo a physical and mental evaluation to emphasize that such ritual surveillance is the duty of those of us who care for others. To make that examination a preliminary requirement for acceptance to medical school risks excluding many who might prove to be very good doctors. Drug and alcohol addiction head the list of potential problems that these checkups could detect—followed by failing mental vigor in aging physicians—but even physical and mental changes as mild as "burnout" can detract from the care of patients. The mental impairment of younger physicians with other chronic conditions also deserves more attention than it has received. In the urge to protect our colleagues, few have seriously discussed what kind of surveillance is in order for *all* physicians.

We think it prudent for physicians to undergo repeated surveys at regular intervals: right after graduation, at the time of board certification, and every 5 years thereafter during an active career. Such surveillance should include an evaluation of emotional and mental status along with a complete general examination.

Physicians must learn to accept the duty of dealing with impaired colleagues and bringing them to attention if necessary, just as they have learned the importance of hard work and fairness in the care of their patients. In addition, we each have a duty to be examined ourselves, even when we feel well or deny that we are sick.

Sick doctors learn new lessons when we lose control over our bodies and our lives. We learn how grateful patients are for physicians who are with them in their troubles. Immigrants to the nation of patients, sick doctors are grateful for minor details, for the kindness of strangers turned friends and caretakers. We become aware of the lack of privacy in the hospital, of the side effects of the drugs that help, and of how wonderful it is that in their new fervor for quality improvement, medical personnel now strive to be kind as well as efficient.

The powerlessness and loneliness of patienthood remind sick doctors of what in health we may have given up: close relationships with our family and friends, time for contemplation, many of the joys of living. In return, we have been blessed with the chance to help others and to earn the spiritual arrogance that comes from doing good.

Most important, sick doctors learn the hard way that a doctor without patients is no doctor at all.

The Other Side of the Bed Rail

MARY O'FLAHERTY HORN, MD

I had certainly been in large medical centers before; there was no reason to feel overwhelmed. I myself am a well-trained internist from a large university—I knew the scene—but this summer morning was different. I was tired and scared. Just 2 weeks before, I had been told that the slurred speech that had been progressing for several months was probably caused by amyotrophic lateral sclerosis (ALS). They'd said 2 to 5 years, and as a physician I knew all too well the grim prognosis and disheartening lack of effective therapy associated with my diagnosis. At the urging of my family, I had come almost 2000 miles to receive a second opinion, but first, I had to undergo electromyography.

Again, I was no stranger to this uncomfortable test. I didn't look forward to the procedure, which Dr. L. would perform before my visit with the consulting neurologist, but I knew it was necessary, and I was resolute. My husband—a schoolteacher with little knowledge of physicians and hospitals except through me—accompanied me to the office. To my dismay, however, he was not allowed to go in with me.

It was apparent on first introduction that Dr. L. was distant. His "Good morning" had an automatic quality about it, and my attempts to make pleasant conversation quickly faltered. He was aware that I was a physician but knew nothing else about me and made it clear that he had no further interest. I lapsed into silence until the residents came in to watch him do the test. As I lay on the table in my gown that barely reached my knees, I summoned what dignity I still possessed and greeted them. They seemed kind, and I was relieved to have them there.

The effect of their presence on Dr. L.'s demeanor was immediate. Suddenly, I was the vehicle for teaching these students about motor-neuron pathology. He addressed all comments to them. I might not have been present except for the obvious need for my muscles. His enthusiasm about the array of abnormal findings was clear as he lectured the students on the "classic findings in ALS." He positively bubbled with joy at finding even more evidence of the sickened state of my motor neurons. If I moved or said that the needle he placed in a muscle was uncomfortable, I was regarded with polite but cool irritation, as though an experimental preparation were not behaving in the expected manner. At one point, as I tried to comply with his requests, my gown rose above my hips. As I reached down to correct the problem, he snapped, "Don't move!" One of the students, taking pity on me, offered a blanket, which I accepted gratefully. The students seemed uncomfortable but remained quiet, and after a grueling 1.5 hours, the procedure was at last finished. Dr. L. marched out of the room, followed by the students, except for one who stopped to wish me well.

As I dressed, I had two immediate thoughts. The first was to escape now and never return, although I hadn't yet met the consultant I'd traveled so far to see. The second was, "Thank God I knew I had ALS before I came in here because this would be the cruelest way to find out." I managed to keep from crying until I stood with my husband in the lobby and his innocent question of "How was it?" came crashing down on me. As I demanded that he take me home then and there, barely able to speak between the sobs, I was regarded with indifference by those in the office.

We stayed after all. My husband's cool head and support prevailed, and the consultant lived up to his billing as a kind and intelligent clinician. But I wondered, "How many patients would have left without getting the care they needed? How often do we treat our patients this way? What did that teach those young residents about the importance of treating patients with empathy and compassion?"

Had I been my usual self, I would not have tolerated such callousness. But when you are sick, the strength and reserves for fighting such treatment are not there. Later, as I mulled over the possibility of taking action, I found that in the press of struggling with a desperate disease, I was still incapable of it. The best I could do was contrast that experience with the kindness and caring that my own physicians provided.

It is a lesson in healing. Although my physicians may not be able to cure my illness, their encouragement, time, patience, and trust build bridges that enable me to cope one day at a time. Encounters such as mine with Dr. L., the antithesis of caring, could become more common as medical care becomes more fragmented and long-term relationships with patients become relics. Physicians are the vital human link that can give patients the strength they require. As the pace of change in medicine quickens, physicians who teach will bear a special responsibility to provide strong examples of empathy and professionalism to students and residents. After all, one day we may all find ourselves on the other side of the bed rail, and those young physicians will become what we model for them today.

Note: Doctor Horn died at home on 10 August 1998. Peter V. Barrett, MD, revised the manuscript after her death.

The Patient as Physician

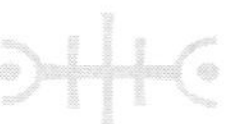

HERBERT S. WAXMAN, MD

The physician who becomes a patient has a chance to become a better doctor. In 1985, I developed sudden chest pain, which led to cardiac catheterization. My physicians found a type I acute aortic dissection, and emergency surgery quickly followed. The cardiopulmonary bypass time was very long, and I received hundreds of units of blood products to maintain hemostasis. After surgery, I sustained extensive lower-extremity necrosis of muscle and nerve, probable deep venous thrombosis, cardiac arrhythmias, total global amnesia, painful peripheral neuropathy, and severe depression. It took me 3 months after the surgery to begin the transition back to my responsibilities as a department chairman and clinician-educator. And I still worry about the longer-term consequences.

Dedicated physicians from many specialties saved my life, for which I have the most profound gratitude. Yet, I learned hard lessons from my experience. Three aspects of my own care are particularly instructive.

Time

After the first 10 days or so, it seemed that my short-term survival was no longer in doubt. As a consequence, my physicians did not have to spend as much time attending to the many details of my medical care. But at the same time, I became preoccupied with questions, concerns, and anxieties. Yet, like most patients, I was hesitant to impose upon my busy physicians. And so, like those of most patients, my anxieties persisted and my questions went unanswered. Later, it came to me: how vital it is that the physician should be sensitive to the possibility that such patient concerns are lying beneath the surface and should fulfill all of his or her patient's needs. Because being a patient means being dependent and vulnerable, the physician needs to take the initiative in asking the patient about unanswered questions or unresolved issues.

Honesty

Later in my course, the dominant clinical issues shifted from the vascular to the neurologic. A painful peripheral neuropathy, probably a consequence of earlier ischemic nerve damage, led to my increasing dependence on analgesics and my diminished capacity for rehabilitation. Consultants were everywhere. There were no ready solutions. Each physician communicated to me the expected natural history of this distressing, if not life-threatening, problem. However, as reassuring as each physician was individually, the information being transmitted differed from physician to physician. As a patient, I could only conclude that lack of knowledge was being masked by communication that probably went beyond the facts. I began to trust my physicians less. Only when another consultant told me that no good information about long-term prognosis was available but that therapeutic options existed that might help did I find myself in the hands of someone whose honesty I could trust. All my physicians were caring and well-intentioned, yet their reluctance to say "I don't know" shook my trust in them.

Recognition of Depression

Several months after the surgery, I developed the most distressing symptoms of all: dysphoria, early morning awakening, joylessness, and a profound sense of unworthiness. I had developed major depression. Yet my physicians did not recognize it and advised me to keep busy and not dwell on the symptoms. Their advice was well-intentioned but, not surprisingly, ineffective. Finally a consultant (and friend) recognized the correct diagnosis. Antidepressants and psychiatric care helped immensely. I could sleep again, make decisions, feel confident, and find a sense of purpose. I learned firsthand that there are two characteristics of depression: It is very painful, and it is treatable. Failure to diagnose it results in failure to institute therapy; as a consequence, the patient continues to suffer. My case was not uncommon. The literature abounds with documentation of the lack of sensitivity of usual primary care to the diagnosis of depression.

* * * *

As I returned to work and to the care of my patients, I found myself dealing with their problems in the context of the illness from which I was recovering. More often than before, I would ask myself three questions, which I was thoroughly convinced were important: Am I allowing enough time to talk to each patient and assess whether there has been an adequate opportunity for questions to have been addressed and concerns relieved? Am I being honest in communicating to each patient what I know but also what I *don't* know in response to his or her questions and concerns? Am I sufficiently sensitive to symptoms of depression (or other treatable psychological and psychiatric conditions) and thereby losing no opportunity to diminish the patient's suffering?

Sadly, I realize that my own sensitivity as a physician differed between the 17 years of practice before my illness and the period thereafter. Unquestionably, my experiences as a patient changed my behavior as a physician. Although I had always thought of myself as a capable, caring internist and hematologist, my medical education had not prepared me to care for patients as well as did the added experience of having myself been a patient. How might it have been otherwise? It is hardly practical to require that every physician have a serious illness as part of the process of preparing to care for patients. (However, many schools now offer opportunities for students to participate in experiences as simulated patients in a real medical environment.) It may prove helpful, however, to listen carefully to physicians who have been patients.

The Genie in the Bottle

MICHAEL BERNSTEIN, MD

In the fall of 1992, my 1-year-old granddaughter developed classic erythema infectiosum. Her face took on the typical "slapped cheek" appearance, and she developed fever and malaise. I suspected that her parvovirus B19 would in all likelihood infect her grandfather, and it did: I developed fever and severe joint pains. Even after these symptoms disappeared, however, I felt poorly and could never seem to recover from an increasing sense of fatigue that persisted and even worsened. In 6 weeks, my hemoglobin concentration decreased to 10 g (possibly due to the parvovirus), and I lost 22 pounds. I had no appetite, despite my wife's best efforts to provide me with my favorite dishes. I simply could not eat more than several hundred calories a day.

I was hospitalized with a working diagnosis of possible pancreatic cancer. I was cachectic and extremely weak. The only clinical finding other than the recent weight loss was a systolic blood pressure of 80 mm Hg, which responded to vigorous hydration. This prompted a very astute clinician to think that the problem might be metabolic, and he called for a cortisol level. It came back at just about zero. Several studies later, an enlarged sella with a 2.5-cm mass was diagnosed and I was prepared for a transphenoidal hypophysectomy.

During this time, my missing hormones were replaced and I developed a ferocious appetite. But as I was celebrating the joys of food, I began to lose vision in my left eye. This was frightening, and none of my physicians were able to reassure me that it would not be permanent. Before my surgery, I quietly began to make "deals" with the Deity. Most of them, surprisingly, did not involve my survival but instead were concerned with my rapidly failing eyesight.

The neurosurgery was successful, and a large, friable, hemorrhagic, benign adenoma was removed. Because of bony erosion, the sella floor was rebuilt. When I awoke, my vision had miraculously returned. The neurosurgeon explained that the mass had been pressing on my left optic nerve. My physicians then transferred me to the intensive care unit, where I was lashed to the bed by three intravascular lines, a catheter, and several chest leads and monitors.

Despite wonderful nursing, I began to lose my sense of night and day. With two enormous nasal drains (which resembled small trumpets) installed, I looked and felt like Miss Piggy, the porcine starlet of *The Muppet Show*. My neurosurgeon stressed the importance of my torso and head remaining upright for several days to let the newly created floor of the sella meld. New fears crept in. Did I have postoperative diabetes insipidus? Was the tumor really benign? Was I developing a cerebrospinal fluid leak? If I slept with my head tilted, would my new sella floor fall off? Irrational, yes, but specific fears that only a physician could conjure up.

Although my family, physicians, and nursing staff were very caring, my real-time 24-hour companion was the television set. I had never realized how important that much-maligned device is to a bedridden patient. It shut down once, shortly after midnight, and had it not been rapidly repaired, the loss would have been akin to that of a close relative. The early hours of the morning can be very lonely.

After several days, I was transferred to the neurosurgical floor and the drains were removed from both nasal passages. I began to feel very lucky and became quite optimistic. The battle had been won. Thanks to modern medicine and surgery, I was happily anticipating my return to work and my resumption of a fairly normal life. But this was not to be.

Several weeks after I was discharged, I returned to work. My physical world then started to come apart. I was extremely fatigued to the point of severe nausea for many hours during the day and into the evening. The exhaustion was similar to what I had experienced as an intern when I went without sleep for 36 or more hours; now, however, I slept several hours a night yet never felt refreshed. Opening jars and bottles became impossible for me. Carrying anything of significant weight was beyond my ability. The stairs to the garage and basement became increasingly difficult to negotiate, and concentrating and retaining information required tremendous mental work. I tried an exercise program, under supervision, but was unable to sustain even the simplest regimen. I could not sit and play with my granddaughter for more than 10 or 15 minutes at a time. I realized that I was clinically, severely depressed. This went on for months without any remission, despite treatment with antidepressants and continued attempts at graded exercise. I was devastated! Although I was in my mid-sixties, I felt like a frail octogenarian.

Finally, during an executive committee meeting at the department of medicine at Columbia University, one of the senior endocrinologists told me that what I was experiencing had been well documented: I probably needed growth hormone. I was stunned. Growth hormone was for children with growth problems. How could lack of a hormone that diminishes naturally with age possibly be causing these crippling symptoms?

With great trepidation and very little faith, I applied for enrollment in a double-blind study of patients without growth hormone. Initial provocative testing revealed that I was an acceptable participant. After instructions from the test team, I began injecting myself with what was either a placebo or actual growth hormone. Within 3 weeks I knew I had drawn the bottle with the "genie": The nausea disappeared. In 3 more weeks, I was once again able to open jars and bottles. My ability to read and retain material, both professional and recreational, returned completely. I could now sit in a chair or on the floor and play for substantial periods of time with my very active granddaughter. As the months progressed, my strength came back, the depression disappeared entirely, and I felt as if I had regained my rightful age.

That was the most terrible voyage of my life. All of my varied symptoms and serious functional difficulties had one simple cause: complete absence of growth hormone. Happily, I live at a time when basic science and genetic engineering have given me back most of the joy that I thought I had lost forever. Of course, the story of this journey would not be complete without noting that I was extremely fortunate to be working with very sophisticated clinicians and researchers. Without their input, I would not have recognized the syndrome that I was suffering from and would not have been directed to a definitive protocol. I can only hope that increasing awareness of this problem will permit more patients to obtain early diagnoses and definitive therapy and return with dignity to their normal, productive lives.

Insight

MARY E. MOORE, MD, PhD

The problems with my eyes had become alarming. Two and a half years ago I was told I had a posterior vitreous detachment in my left eye that had left me with an eye full of floating debris. Over the past 2 weeks, I had developed a similar problem in my right eye, its onset heralded by flashes of light when I turned my head. I found it almost impossible to focus a microscope on joint-fluid samples, a major inconvenience for a rheumatologist. After a MEDLINE search taught me that retinal damage was possible, I decided to consult a specialist at a large eye hospital in the city. My husband agreed to accompany me.

Outside, the massive, modern hospital was impressive. Inside, it was a different story. The entrance was a short, bare hallway ending at a reception desk. A remarkably unreceptive receptionist answered my request for "Dr. Dareeno" with bored, mechanical responses.

"Second floor. Elevators on the right. Retina services." By this time, my predictable anxiety was affecting my bladder capacity, and I was glad to see, on exiting the elevator, a sign for restrooms.

The ladies' room was depressingly filthy, especially considering that the day was only half over. Used paper littered the floor. I had the wild fantasy of sightless women going to the bathroom and washing their hands, all the while flinging dirty toilet paper and towels toward unseen receptacles.

My destination was a cavernous, dimly lit hall, painted a sickly tan, running along one side of the building. It was lined with chairs and potted palms and was punctuated along its inner wall by counters announcing different services. One of the first, and least promising, was "Low Vision." We thankfully left that behind. "Retina Services" was at the far end. I gave my name at that counter and was relieved to learn that I was expected. A sign posted nearby read, "If your vision has not been taken by a technician within 15 minutes after you arrive, please check with the receptionist."

Good Lord, I thought. After they make off with your vision do you go back to the "Low Vision" station? Or was there one I missed called "No Vision"?

My morbid thoughts were interrupted by the clerk behind the counter, who was looking at me speculatively.

"Are you 65?" she asked.

I, who was only 64 and 2 months, replied emphatically, "No."

"Then sit over there and fill out these forms," she instructed. At last, something on which I could concentrate and that would display my superior grasp of medical paperwork. Under *Occupation* I proudly filled in "physician" and wrote, in the space indicated, a brief (21-word) medical history of my eye problem, using "O.D." and "O.S." to display my knowledge of ophthalmologic terminology.

I had long since finished the forms when the technician assigned to "take" my vision called my name for a turn at the eye chart. Why hadn't I cleaned my contact lenses? Now they would think my vision was worse than it really was. I blinked to try to separate the junk on the lenses from the junk in my eyes. Why did the technician's manner give me the feeling that I was flunking an IQ test? When I had humiliated myself sufficiently, she introduced drops into my eyes, careful to give no clue about the effect they would have. Gradually, a nauseating fog involved my visual world.

"Mary Moore," A voice called out through the fog. "Come in and sit down, Mary," requested a young woman, whom I had never met before, in unexpectedly familiar terms. At least she was smiling, the only smile I had seen anywhere in the hospital. A middle-aged man in a white coat approached. Thank goodness, a colleague.

"I'm Dr. Dareeno," the man announced briskly, avoiding my pleading-for-empathy gaze. "Tell me about your eye problems." I could sense I had to talk fast. I began the first of my 21 words. "Yes, yes," he interrupted impatiently. "You've had floaters and flashing lights. Is that correct?"

"Yes," I replied, avoiding any editorializing. I am a quick learner.

"Put your forehead here," he instructed. Moving around his lights and lenses, he peered into my eyes, all the while addressing cryptic dictation to the young woman. Unconnected phrases were alternatingly frightening and baffling. "Lens opacity." "Stone." "PVD." "Pressure." Finally, one that was reassuring. "Retina normal." The examination then abruptly changed. "Lie down here," he said, indicating an examination table. He began a series of very firm pokes, using a cotton-tipped swab. Was the swab poking into my eyeball? Because of the anesthetic he had applied, I couldn't tell—and he certainly had no intention of informing me. What would he do next? "Sit up," he commanded. "Well," he said, gazing at a point over my head, "there is no retinal damage. So everything is fine. But to play it safe, I'd like to check you again in 1 month."

Not exactly fine, I thought. I still had the vision of someone snorkeling in dirty water. "Is there nothing to be done for these floaters?" I asked timidly.

"No. We could drain the vitreous, but it is very risky and you could lose your sight." He started to turn away. My plan to ask about a procedure I had found described in the *British Journal of Ophthalmology* to treat vitreous floaters with neomydium: yttrium-aluminum-garnet lasers suddenly seemed wildly impractical.

"Thank you," I replied with reflexive politeness. I got off the table and stumbled toward the waiting room. There, the dim outline of my husband appeared, as welcome as a familiar landfall after hours lost at sea.

"Everything all right?" he inquired.

"My retina is fine." I paused to consider. "And I learned a lot."

"About your eyes?"

I took his arm for support. "About being a patient . . . . Let's go home."

For Corrie

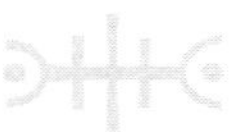

ERIC C. LAST, DO

The birth of our third child was supposed to be a scheduled cesarean section, performed at the hospital where I practice. However, several days before the appointed date, my wife began labor, and her scheduled section turned into an urgent one. Not long after the procedure began, our new baby, our Corrie, was handed to me with the pediatrician's pronouncement, "Here's your perfect baby girl." As I had done twice before, I cradled this new life in my hands as tears of joy and thankfulness welled in my eyes. Too quickly, the circulating nurse took our new angel from me to be officially weighed and measured.

Not more than five minutes later, I felt a hand, gentle yet insistent, on my left shoulder. One of the nurses was there, whispering to me that the pediatrician needed to speak to me. I thought to myself that he was simply being a polite colleague, wanting to wish us luck. Nothing could be wrong, I reasoned, because he had used the words "perfect baby girl." But the look on his face as he waited for me in the hallway told me that something had changed. "I can't be sure," he began haltingly, "but I'm concerned that Corrie may have Down syndrome." He described "some things" that had him concerned, like very low muscle tone and a bothersome transverse crease on her palm. He told me about the tests that would be needed, the specialists who would be called. I shook his hand and thanked him for his thoroughness. I then felt a real physical pain, the likes of which I had never experienced in my life. It began in my gut, went up through my chest, and terminated in a wave of nausea and tremulousness that seized my entire being. I was helped to a chair, given a cup of water, and waited for the obstetrician to complete his work.

Fifteen minutes later, the obstetrician emerged from the OR, looking drawn and shocked. Someone had told him of the events of the preceding minutes, and he immediately came to me and embraced me. Tears again welled up in my eyes, though now they were tears of grief and fear. Once composed, I asked how we were going to give the news to my wife. "That," he began slowly, "is something you are going to have to do." I tried in vain to get someone else, *anyone* else, to give her this piece of news, but all agreed it was best handled by me.

I walked slowly toward the recovery room, the obstetrician's arm around my flagging shoulders. I recalled the many times I had given bad news to patients—news of cancer diagnosed, cancer recurred, AIDS, respiratory failure, any of the awful events that cause the body to fail. I wished I could be back in any of those situations, not to have to complete this task. I took a deep breath, entered the room, and held my wife's hand. "There might be a problem" I said clumsily. "The pediatrician thinks Corrie might have Down syndrome." My wife squeezed my hand, grimaced, and turned her head away. Within minutes she was asleep again, momentarily escaping our new nightmare.

After spending a few moments in the delivery room lounge trying to summon some strength, I somehow made my way downstairs to the doctors' lounge I had been in so many times before. I stared at the familiar phones, knowing I needed to pick one up and start dialing all the loved ones waiting anxiously to hear our good news. But the news I gave wouldn't be good. The hardest call was to our two older kids, telling them (with voice disguised as best I could) about their new sister, who was waiting to see them. I managed to complete the call, hang up the phone, and broke down once again.

I returned to the Nursery, where a pediatric geneticist was present, clipboard-toting assistant at his side, to catalog all of Corrie's parts. He rattled off a list of anomalies that were indicative of the presence of an extra chromosome. Yet, for each one, my brain jumped (ecstatically!) to another family member who had a similar trait. And with each I became convinced that this was all an overreaction, doctors once again looking for things that weren't really there. Yet, there was also a small voice in the back of my head reminding me about zebras and hoofbeats. I knew that I didn't want to believe that something so awful, so strange, could be wrong with our child. Yet, I was starting to believe that they could be right.

The remainder of the first 2 days of Corrie's life were filled with new anxieties. There was difficulty obtaining blood for chromosome studies. Then there was the possibility of a cardiac problem, heralded by cyanosis whenever she cried. There were moments of solace, of comforting words and positive thoughts from colleagues, perspective-building words from the social worker. But there was also a fellow physician who sank beneath insensitivity, gloatingly telling how his wife had an amniocentesis with each pregnancy. "Don't you know you could have terminated if she had an amnio," he asked. Don't you realize (I thought) you are talking about my very real, very alive baby?

Each day I wandered the hallways of the hospital living each of Kubler-Ross's stages. Bargaining was the most interesting. I saw the pediatric ICU ambulance arrive from our affiliated teaching hospital. I thought how much nicer it would be if Corrie had an acute, life-threatening problem, where her future would hinge on some miracle of diagnostic acumen or surgical prowess, where the odds might be heavily stacked against her, but where her life would be forever normal if the procedure were a success. Instead, we had the possibility of a future filled with unknowns, and that unknown void would stretch out for the rest of Corrie's life, and of ours.

Beyond the shock and fear, the overriding feeling during that first week was that something very special had been stolen from us. There were little things that should have happened, but couldn't. The expectations of all the happy visits and handshakes in the hospital now turned into looks of sadness, expressions of condolence. There were the walks to the nursery, gazing at all of the newborns, and staring at Corrie, trying to convince myself that she looked no different from the others. There was the traditional "surf and turf" dinner for new parents the night before discharge, when my wife and I went through the motions of enjoying ourselves, unable to hide our anxieties or sadness from each other.

One week after Corrie's birth, the geneticist called to say that yes the results were in and yes there were three #21 chromosomes. But the real impact of that news didn't really hit until I saw the actual karyotype, with perfectly symmetrical rows of chromosome pairs except above the number 21, where an extra piece of genetic material lay waiting to change our family's life forever.

It is now a year since Corrie's birth, and our lives truly have been changed, changed in ways I could not have imagined 12 months ago. No longer do I think of words like "horror" and "fear" when I describe our situation, or her life. I think of the beautiful images I have seen: the joyful expression on my wife's face that has replaced her dread, the sheer delight our older children get when Corrie responds to their play, the look (that I'm convinced she reserves for me) Corrie gets when her daddy holds her, the incredible joy we all feel as she attains each milestone. I think of the progress she has made, and of the staff of teachers and therapists who have cared for her, and who have, for me, defined the word "dedication."

And yes, she has changed the way I live, and so has changed the way I practice medicine. I have a new sense of appreciation for my truly ill patients, and maybe a little less patience for those with trivial complaints. I have seen unbelievable coincidences in my practice, such as the friendship of a man I have cared for over the past 6 years whose family has adopted a series of children with Down syndrome, or the grandmother who came into my office bursting with pride 2 years before Corrie's birth telling me of her grandson's Bar Mitzvah, her grandson with Down syndrome. I have drawn strength from so many, including one patient, dying of AIDS, who knew of our situation and who cared enough to ask.

But mostly I think I have learned about myself, and about love. And while we don't know what the future will hold for Corrie, I realize we can't predict this for anyone, even for ourselves. I realize that I have made certain foolish assumptions in my life. I took it as a given that my children would all go to school, would all attain some stature in the world that I used to know, and take for granted. But that world is very different to me now, and I realize just how arrogant such assumptions really are. And because of that, I have learned to try to appreciate all that surrounds me, as often as I can, for there is truly so much to be amazed by, and to be thankful for.

Health Care in America: An Intimate Glimpse

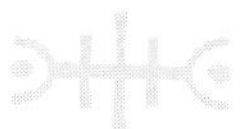

BYRON FARWELL

I am an obese 75-year-old man. I recently had a large cyst removed from my spine, along with some bits of bone for which the surgeon said I had no need. The surgeon, trained at the University of Pennsylvania and Harvard, had an impressive résumé and came highly recommended. He was, in addition, a very likable fellow. He looked about 18 years old.

I had last had surgery 30 years earlier in Switzerland, where I had a large room with a window overlooking the Alps in a hospital that boasted a splendid wine cellar. The nurses, efficient and caring, even brought drinks for visitors. When I experienced a bit of postoperative trauma, the surgeon was at my bedside within minutes with a sizable glass of cognac. I speculated recently on how patients were now cared for, more than a quarter of a century later, in the United States, my native land. Rather differently, I discovered.

The operation itself, as far as I could tell, went very well. I had naively assumed that I would have a private room, but perhaps all of them were occupied; it was not offered as an option. I awoke to find myself on a narrow bed in a small room that I shared with another patient. A curtain separated me from my fellow sufferer, whom I never saw. He enjoyed the window overlooking the parking lot. I was able to note his television preferences, which were limited to cartoons and basketball. I also saw his many friends and relations of both sexes and all ages, who, perforce, had to squeeze past my bed to reach the toilet, of which they seem to have had frequent need.

The room was stuffy and uncomfortable. Although the weather was not inclement, the window remained fast shut; not a whiff of fresh air was admitted. In Britain during the mid-19th century, a scandal arose when it was learned that the standard for soldiers' barracks was only 800 cubic feet of air per man. I mentally tried to gauge the amount of air space available to me. Not that much, I reckoned.

My new habitat was a world of women: registered nurses, practical nurses, nurses' aides, student nurses, technicians, cleaning women, and women who brought and removed trays of food. Most of the nurses were saints. Certainly they were during my first night after surgery, when neither the do-it-yourself painkiller kit with which I was provided nor the shots of who-knows-what narcotic relieved my "discomfort"—the physician's word for excruciating pain. A brave nurse dared wake the surgeon at midnight, and the surgeon kindly increased the dosages of painkillers so that they eventually brought me relief.

The next day, my do-it-yourself painkiller was removed from me. When told what was to replace it, I expressed doubts to the nurse about its efficacy, for it had been tried before my operation without success. To my astonishment, she reacted as if I had personally insulted her. (Is the nurses' pension fund invested in a pharmaceutical company?) She roughly removed all the tubes from my wrist and slapped on a bandage. As she dismantled the gadget from which the bags hung, she said, "*I'm* not going to reinsert this." And with that she marched out.

Within minutes blood oozed from my wrist, then gushed. I rang for a nurse, but when no one responded, I hailed a nurse passing by in the hall. (There was, I discovered, an advantage in having a bed by the door rather than the window.) She grabbed a sheet, bound my wrist, and dispatched an aide to fetch proper bandages. She did her job efficiently and then cleaned up the bed, by now thoroughly blood soaked. A real saint. I do not know that my regular nurse was made aware of this incident.

Food at the hospital was provided by cooks who had failed to qualify as airline chefs. No salt was allowed, and the hospital appeared ignorant of salt substitutes. It scarcely mattered. The food was served tepid at best, arrived at odd hours, and always appeared unappetizing, except to the resident fly who seemed to find dried baked beans with a piece of desiccated turkey delicious. I ate only some fruit. No one noticed whether I ate or not. I suppose it was an added bonus if I lost a few pounds.

I was never cleaned up. When I felt well enough to clean myself, I requested a wash rag and hand towel. I thus managed to scrub off some of the dried blood and remnants of adhesive tape.

The major concern of the staff was to see that I urinated—or, to use the medical term favored by the nurses, "peed." Nurses propped me up beside the bed and held out a urinal, asking me if I could perform. Standing between two young women who watched carefully, I said I thought not. As I found myself unable to provide urine under any circumstance, a catheter was inserted in my penis. However uncomfortable and dignity-deflating this procedure seemed, it was done quickly and professionally. Such was not the case the second time.

It was hands-on day for the local nursing school, and fresh-faced young female students came to take my blood pressure, feel my pulse, and stick needles in my buttocks. I was no longer a mere patient but a warm body on which budding Florence Nightingales could practice. Any remnant of human dignity I possessed was shredded when a pretty teenager was called on to insert a catheter. The student and her tutor bent over the bed to examine my genitalia in detail. The student appeared never to have seen such a sight and handled my penis gingerly while her instructor explained the organ and what she was supposed to do with it. I had become an exhibit in a sex education class.

When the time came for me to be discharged, a nurse or an aide (impossible to tell which since nurses stopped dressing like nurses) held up a plastic basin full of toilet articles—a small tube of toothpaste and a toothbrush, a bottle of baby powder, a small plastic comb, and other items, with a total worth of about $12—and asked if I wanted them. When I said I had never seen them before, she brightly replied, "Yer payin' for 'em."

She was right. When the first bill came, I was charged $890.20 for "pharmacy." Of course, a few other items were included, as I noticed when I received an itemized bill, perhaps, all told, as much as $40 at hospital prices. Hospital bills are difficult for the uninitiated to read, filled as they are with abbreviated, arcane medical terms. But I did see allopurinol on the list. I was charged $1.45 for one allopurinol pill (local retail price, 2.4 cents), a medicine effective only for gout. Actually, the bill listed four pills, but three, perhaps in a spasm of guilt, had been removed.

In the automobile business, such practices are called "add-ons." Car dealers who try this stunt often end up in court. How does a hospital get away with it? Not long ago, *The Washington Post* carried an article on credit card companies that had to pay the Federal Trade Commission $292,000 because they charged people for services they had never agreed to buy. Has no former hospital patient, I wondered, ever complained to the FTC?

It was like returning home from another planet when at last I was discharged. It was still a female world, but it was inhabited by a loving wife and our two tail-wagging dogs. It was a familiar world, a comfortable world, with fresh air, edible food, and a drink in a large chair before the fire, where I could contemplate the problems of health care in America and deplore the cost of airline tickets to Switzerland.

A Letter from a Patient's Daughter

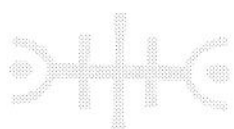

ELISABETH HANSOT, PHD

My mother, Georgia Hansot, died recently in the intensive care unit of a major hospital in the eastern United States. She was 87 years old. This is an account of the 5 days she spent in the hospital from the point of view of her daughter, a 57-year-old professional woman who was charged with her mother's power of attorney for health care. My intent is to convey the experience of one person thrust into the unfamiliar world of hospital routines and intensive care units. My mother's experience died with her; I can describe only what I experienced and what I understood her to be trying to communicate.

This essay could as easily be entitled "There Are No Villains Here." Medical personnel, trained to save lives and not to let patients die, exerted themselves to that end. Hospital staff and the families of other patients in the intensive care unit, as time and ability allowed, tried to comfort. Nonetheless, those 5 days were among the loneliest and most disorienting that I have ever experienced.

As I think back on it, I am astounded that I had so little inkling of how hard it would be to help my mother have the death she wanted. A widow of 6 years, my mother had retained the no-nonsense attitude of her Kansan farming origins. She lived in an affluent and stable community on the east coast, and she saw her physician of

25 years routinely for checkups. When we talked together about how she wanted to die, she was clear, consistent, and matter-of-fact. She hoped for a swift death and wanted no unnecessary prolongation of her life.

Entrusted with a general power of attorney and a power of attorney for health care, I believed that I could make decisions on her behalf as she would want them made if she were to become incapacitated. As it turned out, I was woefully unprepared for what was in store for her and for me.

On a spring morning in April, my mother abruptly became ill and was promptly admitted to the local hospital. When I arrived in the late afternoon, she was resting comfortably after a long day of diagnostic tests. Because she had been tired by the day's ordeal, I stayed only briefly, promising to be back early in the morning with newspapers and books. I left my number with the nurse, in case of an emergency.

At 2 o'clock the next morning, I was awakened by a call from the night nurse. My mother had suddenly taken a turn for the worse and was being transferred to intensive care. I arrived on the hospital floor just as the gurney was being wheeled into the unit. My mother's face was covered by an oxygen mask, but she was able to respond to my voice with an exclamation. It was the last time she would be able to do so.

I tried to accompany her into the intensive care unit but could not. The physician in charge firmly instructed me to stay outside until my mother was "taken care of." An hour later, when I was allowed to see her, she was attached to a respirator and had a feeding tube inserted down her throat.

What had happened? My mother had left a carefully updated power of attorney for health care with her physician, her lawyer, and her offspring, reaffirming her determination not to have her life prolonged by artificial means. Exactly the opposite of what she had wished had occurred; the living will had become invisible just when it was needed most. My mother's physician, it turned out, had not notified the medical team of her advance directive, and the hospital, despite a 1990 federal law that mandates such inquiries, did not ask my mother whether she had such a document. And I, in turn, had neglected to check that the physicians and nurses knew about her desire not to have heroic measures used to prolong her life.

Over the ensuing 5 days, I came to understand how serious the results of these omissions were. I found that I was dealing with a bewildering array of medical specialists trained to prolong lives, not to let patients die. During the first day that my mother was in the intensive care unit, I asked her physician to make it clear to the attending medical personnel that she had given me durable power of attorney for health care. He readily complied. I was told that my mother had had a stroke and that she would not recover from her hemiparalysis. The physicians hoped to fit her with a tracheostomy tube and send her to a nursing home. From my many conversations with my mother about quality of life and medical care, I knew that she did not want such a life. Yet my mother's wishes, as they were understood by her family physician and her daughter, were now subject to the approval of strangers: the cadre of cardiologists, neurologists, and pulmonologists who attended her.

None of these specialists knew my mother, and they all had their convictions about how to do best by her. Most notably, they varied in the latitude with which they were willing to interpret her wishes (I had become her spokesperson; my only sibling, an older brother, was out of the country). The variance was widest between my mother's wishes and those of the attending pulmonologist: He made it clear that his approach was conservative in such matters. He found it nearly impossible to accept that my mother would prefer death to living with hemiparalysis and a tracheotomy. Over the next several days, our conversations became terser and tenser as he raised such questions as whether perhaps I was an ageist, or an ideologue interested only in abstract principles. I asked the family physician whether another pulmonologist could attend the case, only to be told that all of the pulmonologists accredited to the hospital shared similar beliefs.

My stress built over the ensuing 5 days as my mother's distress was palpable. She successfully tore out her feeding tube only to have it reinserted and her restraints tightened. An attempt to remove my mother from the ventilator failed; her swollen larynx prevented her from breathing on her own. I had agreed to the removal on the condition that I be allowed to stay with her during the attempt. Afterward, the pulmonologist declared himself pleased that he had been able to reinsert her breathing tube, barely in time. He seemed, however, unaware of how agitated this process had left her. I asked that she be sedated, and an obliging nurse obtained permission for this.

The hospital increasingly came to feel like alien territory, full of medical strangers intent on maintaining my mother's vital signs at all costs. During her ordeal, my mother became increasingly frantic. She continually leaned against her restraints, trying to get her hand close enough to her feeding tube to tear it out again. My sense of being trapped in a nightmare intensified.

In the long days that I spent with her, I learned to read her increasing anguish through her refusals to have her mouth swabbed or to have the secretions in it suctioned dry. One afternoon, she rapped her cuffed hand angrily against the bed bars to get my attention, then motioned toward the tubes that she clearly wished to have removed. The next day, when I was holding her hand, she squeezed mine so hard that I winced in pain, and after that a breakthrough came: We were able to devise a mode of talking to each other.

In response to a yes or no question, my mother nodded or shook her head. Once this mode of communication was clearly established, I was able to ask my mother twice—with her nurse as a witness, and with 4 hours between each question—whether she wished to die. My very clearheaded and determined mother thus was able, finally, to assert herself for the necessary last time. The nurse informed the physicians of what she had seen. Then the wait began. The hours dragged by as the specialists were persuaded, one by one, to give their consent. Finally, a technician was allowed to pull the tube from my mother's throat. None of the physicians who had attended her was present.

In retrospect, as I review the events of those painful 5 days, there seems to be no simple explanation for what happened. Physicians are trained to save lives, and most of us would not have it otherwise. In their conversations with me, my mother's physicians related success stories: A paralyzed man with his faculties intact had lived a full decade longer with a tracheostomy; a woman (the mother-in-law of one of the physicians) with a condition similar to my mother's was still alive to that day, semiparalyzed, in a nursing home. I asked this physician whether he thought his mother-in-law was satisfied with this outcome. He responded, honestly enough, that he did not know.

These stories were intended to be helpful, to open up for me possibilities beyond the intensive care unit. But in the end they turned into so many cautionary tales. Most of the stories seemed to define success as survival and ended with the patient's departure from the hospital. The quality of life after that departure was, at best, moot. Everything I knew about my mother made me certain that she did not desire to continue her life in a semiparalyzed condition.

Subsequently, I wondered if the fact that so many physicians attended my mother may have restrained any one of them from helping me figure out how to be effective on her behalf. After all, critical care physicians must work with each other day in and day out. The cost of challenging the judgment or sensibilities of any member of the medical team must be high indeed. Any single case, by contrast, is a brief bird of passage.

In the weeks that followed my mother's ordeal, I listened, with the rest of the United States, to accounts of the deaths of Richard Nixon and Jacqueline Onassis. Because both of them had living wills, the commentators explained, their lives would not be prolonged by mechanical means. Angry and frustrated at the way my mother had died, I wondered: Do you have to be notable to be heard in our society?

All told, I think that my mother was fortunate. In the long run, her wishes were followed; 5 days in the intensive care unit compares favorably with the experiences of many other elderly persons. But the experience was harrowing, for her and for me. What is routine for hospital staff is all too often the first experience of its kind for critically ill patients and their families. I had a very steep and painful learning curve. This essay is written in the hope that hospitals will devise procedures so that patients and their families can, with less pain and perplexity than I experienced, decide when and how death arrives.

A Reluctant Doctor Shopper

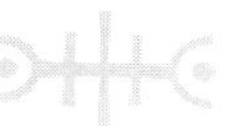

JUNE BINGHAM

A healthy septuagenarian, I found myself on a Monday night dreaming that I was fainting. I woke up and *was* fainting.

On Tuesday, I forgot a lunch date for the first time in my life. That night, I again dreamed that I was fainting—and was.

On Wednesday, I wondered whether to engage in my regular tennis game. "Oh well," I thought. "When in doubt, exercise." Afterward, to my surprise, I felt much peppier and less forgetful.

On Thursday, however, while walking the dog, I had to sit down on a rock and put my head between my knees. Even so, I nearly passed out.

When I got home, I phoned my internist and described the symptoms. In addition to the black scrim descending in front of my eyes, I had the sensation that a cape of ice was being laid across my shoulders, with the chill descending to both elbows. The internist said that the problem sounded neurologic and gave me the name of a specialist to call. I called, but the neurologist could not see me until the following Monday.

On Friday, the frequency of the attacks increased; Saturday, even more so. For the first time in all the years that my internist and I have been together, I phoned him at home to ask whether the tennis that had proved so beneficial on Wednesday might now actually be dangerous. He was in the shower, but his teenager took the message. He never called back.

By early afternoon, I was miserable and phoned a friend, a retired internist. "Doesn't sound neurologic to me," he said. "Call your cardiologist." The cardiologist was out of town at a meeting, but his colleague would get in touch with me. Some 6 hours later, the colleague phoned and told me to go immediately to the emergency department.

Once there, I was wired for sound and sent to a heart monitoring floor. By then, it was 2:30 A.M. Just before 7 A.M., the two residents who had cared for me the night before burst into the room, their young faces alight. "We've got it!"

"Got what?"

"What's wrong with you."

"Oh. What?

"Your heart stops."

"Oh."

Later that day, I was moved to the cardiac intensive care unit because the staff there had more experience with external pacemakers. I was in my cubicle, with my husband sitting by my bed, when I said that I felt another episode coming on.

As I spoke, he turned toward the heart monitor. His face went pale, and he raced from the room. I looked up at the monitor. Absolutely flat. Not a ripple. Wait a minute, I thought. I'm dead, but I'm observing it, too.

My husband had a much harder time. At the central section of the intensive care unit, he grabbed the first physician he saw. "Help," he said, "my wife's in trouble." The physician looked at the number of my cubicle. "Not my patient." Then, taking pity, he said, "Look behind you." Out from the nurses' station, at a run, came a technician, a nurse, and a resident. They switched on the current of the external pacemaker, which I didn't like at all.

"Knock it off," I yelled. "I'd rather have the episode."

"No, you wouldn't!" They persisted.

Finally, my cardiologist surfaced and suggested that I spend the rest of Sunday in the intensive care unit. On Monday, I could have a permanent pacemaker.

The physician-wife of my internist also came to the intensive care unit to visit a patient. She popped into our cubicle and explained why I had felt so much better after the tennis: It had provided what my poor oxygen-starved brain was yearning for. She also said that her husband had not thought that any message about tennis was likely to be serious.

A year later, I went to the surgeon for a checkup. I placed a doodad against the left side of my chest while he fiddled with his computer. "What were you doing yesterday at 11 in the morning?" he asked.

I thought a moment. "Tennis."

"Good."

"Why?"

"Your pulse went up to 150."

So here I am, with a chaperone in my chest, an improved tennis game, and a wonderful new internist. Why did I change from my distinguished physician, who is active in both teaching and administration in one of the leading hospitals in the United States?

First, his wrong diagnosis endangered my life and, because there was no warning not to drive, perhaps the lives of others. Second, not returning my phone call further undermined my trust in his medical judgment. After all, I had scrupulously never bothered him at home; he should have known that I would not do so frivolously. Finally, he was too busy to follow up when I was still in the hospital for the post-operative afternoon and night and when I went home.

Should I have phoned and discussed all this with him? I thought about it, but it would have been painful and made my heart pound. I figured that if he was a good doctor, he could figure it out for himself.

What the Book Says

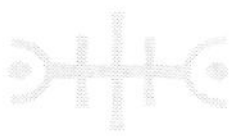

CHAD D. KOLLAS, MD

"May I please have something for pain?"

"Well, I'll have to page the surgical intern on call. Nothing is ordered because you have the epidural."

"Thank you," I called to the nurse as she left the room. The plain, institutional clock below the wall-mounted television read 8:00 P.M. My wife and I chatted idly while sitcoms played in the background. An hour passed. The pain grew worse. I pressed the nurse button on my hospital bed.

"Has the surgical intern ordered anything for pain?"

"Well, he checked the book and paged his senior resident. They said to give you this."

"What is it?"

"Famotidine." The nurse handed me a paper cup of water and the pill. Then she left again.

My wife and I laughed. "I guess you won't get heartburn," quipped my wife.

"I suppose they're giving me this because they gave me an injection of ketorolac yesterday. Oh, well." I took the famotidine.

Another hour passed, and the surgical intern wandered in. "How are you now?"

"The pain is worse than it was."

"My senior resident said that we should wait for a while." The surgical intern turned and walked out.

Great. He probably thinks that I'm seeking narcotic analgesics. I bet he's never had an incision from his xiphoid to his pubis. I guess I'll have to wait it out.

The plain clock stared at me. 10:30 P.M. The pain was worse. The nurse came to check my vital signs. "Your blood pressure is 98/50. Normal."

Normal, unless you consider my history of hypertension and my current pain. Mildly worrisome, actually.

"Excuse me," I interrupted. "Could you please tell me what my last hemoglobin level was?"

"It was 7.1 mg/dL this morning, I think. I told the surgical intern, but he said that the book says you don't need a transfusion."

The book? Oh, yes. I had seen a manual in the surgical intern's pocket when he did my preoperative history and physical. It contained algorithms and information on preoperative preparation and such.

"Thank you."

My preoperative hemoglobin level was 13.6 mg/dL. I had surgery yesterday, and by this morning the hemoglobin level had dropped to 7.1 mg/dL. I bet it's even lower than that now. It sure feels that way—I'm exhausted, even though I'm just lying in bed.

"Could you please page the anesthesia resident on the acute pain service? I'm really in a lot of discomfort. And I think that the surgical intern thinks I'm just seeking more painkillers."

"Sure." The nurse left. My wife looked concerned.

At about 10:45 P.M., the nurse returned. "The anesthesia resident is tied up right now with a pediatric patient. She'll be up here as soon as she can."

"Thank you."

Time passed. I looked at the clock when the pain had become unbearable. 11:30 P.M. The anesthesia resident hurried in, smiling. A new night shift nurse followed. The anesthesia resident quickly checked the pump that controlled the epidural anesthetic. "Oh, I see.

Here's the problem. The line is kinked just inside the pump, but the sensor doesn't sense it. The readout indicates you're getting anesthetic when you're really not. So you've been without analgesia for hours. I'm sorry." I felt vindicated.

See, I told you so.

"I'll need to bolus your epidural catheter with more anesthetic," she continued. "It'll take a few minutes to get it ready. The medication will relieve your pain, but it may cause some hypotension." The surgical intern walked in.

"I think you should know that my hemoglobin level this morning was 7.1 mg/dL," I told the anesthesia resident. "I would bet that it's lower than that now."

"Why haven't they given you some blood?" asked the anesthesia resident as she prepared her syringes.

"Because the book says not to," the irate surgical intern chimed in defensively. "Not unless the hemoglobin level is less than 7.0 mg/dL."

"Please listen to me for a minute," I requested, looking at the surgical intern. "I don't want to tell you how to manage my care, but I'm a little concerned about how things are going right now."

The truth is that I'd like to avoid a catastrophe.

"My surgery ended late yesterday," I continued. "My hemoglobin level 18 hours ago—that is, 12 hours after the surgery—was 7.1 mg/dL. It was 13.6 mg/dL just before that. I'm sure it's even less now. It didn't have a chance to reequilibrate by the time of the last blood draw."

The surgical intern looked blank and unimpressed.

Come on. Listen.

"My Jackson-Pratt drain has also malfunctioned, so blood is leaking out around the drain. No one has measured the blood in the dressings, which the nurses have changed hourly since this morning. I've been taking corticosteroids for more than a year, and you've begun to cut back the stress doses of corticosteroids already. I have a history of hypertension, and my baseline blood pressure runs about 140/80. Now it's—"

The automatic blood pressure cuff promptly beeped and the display read—

"92/58," I added, "even though I'm in a lot of pain. If I were you," I said, watching the surgical intern closely, "I'd strongly consider giving a transfusion now."

Your book just doesn't take the whole clinical picture into account. I know you wouldn't be here if you didn't have some clinical judgment. Please, do what you think is right. Have confidence in yourself.

He paused and thought. "The book says your hemoglobin level has to be less than 7.0 mg/dL before we give you blood," he chanted. My heart sank. "But I'll ask my senior resident what he thinks."

"Thank you." As the surgical intern left, the anesthesia resident fiddled with the epidural pump. "I have to get to the intensive care unit for an emergency, so I'll do this now. I'm going to bolus your epidural."

A few minutes passed. The surgical intern returned. "My senior says the book says no transfusion."

"Would you please at least recheck my hemoglobin level?" I pleaded.

"Okay." He left.

"You should be feeling some relief of your pain now," the anesthesia resident said calmly.

"I am, but I feel a little lightheaded." I glanced at the automatic blood pressure monitor. It read 72/50. I closed my eyes and sank deep into the pillow. I could hear the nurse and the anesthesia resident scurrying about the room. My wife held my hand and squeezed.

Thank God they let her stay past visiting hours.

"Yeah. I definitely don't feel so well." I felt the head of the bed tilting downward. Everything looked dark and fuzzy. I felt so weak.

"Give him a 500-cc bolus of normal saline," the anesthesia resident called out.

"Hang in there, honey," my wife whispered into my right ear.

Then a male voice whispered into my left ear. It was the night nurse. "It's okay. I know how sick you are. I won't let them, the residents, well—you'll be okay."

Great, I can just see it now. The intensive care unit team gathered around my bed. Hypotension leading to acute tubular necrosis and renal failure requiring hemodialysis. Months in the hospital. Just great.

When I finally opened my eyes, the plain, institutional clock read 1:30 A.M.

"Your blood is here," announced the cheerful voice of the night nurse. He winked at me and carried in two units of packed red blood cells. The surgical intern appeared at the base of the bed. As the nurse connected the transfusion bags to my intravenous line, the surgical intern spoke.

"Your last hemoglobin level was down to 6.6 mg/dL. The book said to give you blood."

"Yeah, thanks," I replied weakly. The surgical intern silently hurried out.

I looked over at my wife. She looked exhausted but relieved. "Your blood pressure dropped to 46/20. But it's back up to 92/50 now. Get some rest." I slept.

In the morning, the attending surgeon stopped by, punctual and chipper as usual. "Looks like you got some blood last night."

Yeah. Just like the book said.

Mark Twain's Cat

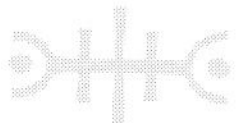

GEORGE M. ANDES

Mark Twain has been credited with the following bit of wisdom: "The boy who carries a cat around by its tail learns a lesson that can be taught in no other way."

Fourteen years ago, I discovered I was holding a cat by its tail. My cat was a great-grandchild of the breed first identified in 1817 by James Parkinson. In the beginning, my cat was a small kitten—a bad-tempered kitten, to be sure, but still just a kitten.

Those of us with a chronic, progressive illness are scarce enough to be objects of mild curiosity but also common enough that everyone knows, or at least knows of, one or more of us. The present bittersweet stage of modern medical science (it is able to prolong life without necessarily restoring health) ensures that, as time passes, more and more people will become like us. I can speak directly only about Parkinson disease, but I suspect that the human condition is sufficiently general that the experiences of those who have diabetes or muscular dystrophy or rheumatoid arthritis or any other chronic ailment will not be greatly misrepresented by my particular experience.

My cat and I have had 14 years of forced companionship but certainly not 14 years of friendship. My unhappy kitten has grown into a large, angry cat. For 14 years, he has hissed at me, spit at me, clawed me, and bitten me. He has slowed my step and stooped my back. He has slurred my speech and caused me to shake. He has stolen my balance and disturbed my sleep. He gives no quarter. When I get angry and give him a good shaking, he becomes furious and spits and lashes out with his claws. When I try to placate him, he bites me. He demands my full attention. If I turn my face away, he claws my ear. My companion's anger is unrelenting, and the damage he does is both progressive and irreversible.

Essayist and PBS [Public Broadcasting System] commentator Richard Rodriguez has correctly observed that education is not at all concerned with improving students' self-esteem. In fact, children enter school with poor skills, limited imaginations, and heads full of wrong facts. They must learn better skills. They must open themselves to the world as it is. They must put away childish notions. They must cast off self-pride and self-esteem. Then they can learn.

My cat does not care about my self-esteem. He gives me lessons in living with adversity and lessons in how to get around and get along with an increasingly useless body, a body that every day is less and less under my voluntary control. My self-esteem is up to me. If I am offended or embarrassed by my cat's latest attack on my dignity, that's my problem.

Here are some of the lessons my cat has taught me, beginning with the most elementary. My family has my Parkinson disease. That was a hard lesson for me to learn. For a long time I resisted the obvious fact that my condition affected others. I selfishly wanted to keep my disease to myself. Finally, thoroughly annoyed at my willful wrong-headedness, my four children told me in no uncertain terms to grow up and get with it. They wanted a father, not a martyr or a sphinx. They wanted me to take them seriously, to talk to them about my disease and myself, and to listen to them when they wanted to talk.

My bonnie Jean, my wife, has my Parkinson disease; she worst of all. As I slowly succumb to my angry cat, she must work ever harder. Her responsibilities increase as my abilities decline. We who carry the cane get attention. They who walk beside us with tired steps, weary faces, and sad eyes, they who care for us, get none. Yet they bear a heavy burden, and they need support and recognition.

I have finally learned to ask for help when I need it. That was a lesson I resisted learning for a long time. It took me several years before I felt easy about asking for absolutely necessary help in opening a door or in putting on a raincoat. I have also learned to be gracious and accept kind offers of help that I may not really need.

Each time I ask for or accept help, I feel little bits and pieces of my independence slipping away. I feel myself drifting from the kingdom of the healthy to the kingdom of the afflicted, from the society of the competent to the society of those who cannot manage by themselves, from the congregation of the normal to the congregation of the not quite normal.

I have learned that things may not be as they first appear. Some time ago, our daughter Mary mentioned to her mother that Dad should have a wheelchair. Jean told her not to be too quick to mention it to me. She guessed, rightly, that I wouldn't hear of it. Shortly thereafter, a friend told me that she thought I should get a wheelchair for those times when I needed one. I said that I didn't want to be wheelchair-bound.

"How about housebound?" she replied. "Is that what you want?" End of argument. If I stubbornly persist in maintaining habits and attitudes that are no longer useful, I neither learn nor prosper. So, foolish pride, get thee behind me. A wheelchair is not the end of the world.

My cat has taught me that I have within me reserves of strength and patience and courage that I would not have thought possible. I have learned that stubbornness and contrariness are virtues. That makes me very virtuous indeed. Every day, my angry cat forcibly impresses on me the fact that without the love and care of others, I am nothing. I also now know that I should never judge the burdens of others by their behavior. We are all very good at looking better than we are; we all carry burdens in private that we prefer to hide in public.

None of us succeed entirely on our own. Success is as much collective as it is individual. My success in remaining useful over the past

14 years has come at least 50% from my stubbornness. I am not modest about that, but by myself I would be nothing. Three headmasters have stood by me and kept me gainfully employed. For 14 years, my faculty colleagues have held me up and tolerated me. They have not coddled me but have held my feet to the fire and kept me honest and made me do my job, yet they have been patient with me and let me be myself. For that, I am grateful beyond words.

I often refer to my Parkinson disease as my peculiar gift. That distresses my family. But I have always accepted my good fortune and many good gifts without complaint and without acknowledgment or thanks. On what grounds, therefore, should I now complain to the Almighty? Please understand me. I do not like my Parkinson disease. It has robbed me of my independence, taken pleasure from my life, stripped away my self-confidence, sapped my energy, depressed my family, separated me from my friends, driven me from my profession, and darkened my future. Yet it has also, as Mark Twain knew, been able to teach me lessons and give me insights that I could have learned in no other way.

As I look back on my education, three teachers, apart from my parents and my children, stand far above the rest: my first-grade teacher, Miss Davis; my wife, Jean; and my angry cat. Each has given me a wonderful gift.

Miss Davis taught me to read and thereby gave me the world of the printed page. Jean's gift to me has been her personal example of integrity in adversity and her polite but uncompromising insistence that women and girls are entitled to and therefore must be given the same rights and privileges and opportunities as men and boys, a view that is not universally held. My cat's gift to me has been the gift of unwelcome truth. He holds before me the mirror of self-revelation and forces me to stare into it, unblinking.

Until I see myself as I am.

Doing Everything

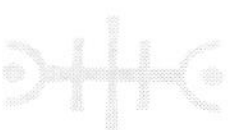

DAVID S. PISETSKY, MD, PHD

I never knew what death was like until I watched my father die. He had Lou Gehrig's disease. I learned about the meanness of this condition only as I saw what it did to him. Until he developed amyotrophic lateral sclerosis at 84 years of age, my father worked full time as a physician and was a robust man with a large belly and an exuberant smile. After he got sick, he became immobile, despondent, and dependent on others. He had difficulty swallowing and, terrified of choking, restricted his diet to soft foods. He lost 100 pounds.

Toward the end of the summer, my mother phoned urgently to tell me that my father's condition had deteriorated. She said that he had suddenly lost the power of speech and refused food and water. I took the first flight out the next morning and speeded from the airport in a rental car. When I arrived at my family's home and saw my father, I was sure that he would die soon. He was in a hospital bed in the living room. He did not respond to my voice. His breathing was rapid and his gaze opaque. I went to the kitchen where my mother sat. She looked anxiously at me. I was now the physician, no longer just the son.

"He's very sick," I said. "What do you want to do?"

"What can I do?" she said. Her eyes were tense, and the tremor that was usually confined to her left hand seemed to seize her whole body.

"We can go to the hospital."

"He hates the ambulance. The sirens scare him. Suppose we don't go?"

"He'll die today."

"So soon?" she said. Her voice was strained. My father was 86 years old and had been miserably sick for 2 years. His death had lurked every day since a fateful electromyogram had led to his diagnosis; nevertheless, its imminence took her by surprise.

"I'll take him myself in the car," I said.

"Thank you," she said, crying. "I'm not ready for him to die."

I went to the living room to get my father. Anyone who says that caring for an old person is like caring for a baby is wrong. The flesh of babies is soft and buoyant. The flesh of old people is dense and dispirited. My father had no muscles. Coarse skin covered bones that were held together by tendons that seemed frayed and rigid. I was afraid that I would pull off a limb if I lifted him wrong.

I put him over my shoulder the way I had been taught to remove hospitalized patients during a fire. I carried him part of the way to the car and stopped so that I could inspect his face. To my horror, he looked dead. In retrospect, I realize that because of the way I was carrying him, he had no venous return and I had put him into shock. I recoiled at the possibility of bringing my own father into an emergency department after he had died in the back seat of a garish red car that smelled of cigarettes.

I carried my father back to his bed and told my mother that he had said he wanted to be at home. "It's better this way. We can all be together."

During the next few hours, my sister, her husband, my niece, and my aunt all came to spend one last day with my father.

"We're all here," my mother said into my father's ear and, for an instant, I thought his head moved in recognition.

"Can he hear?" my aunt asked. My father was her baby brother. They were the last of six siblings. Because I was a physician, she presumed I had knowledge of such mysteries of consciousness.

"I think so," I said with authority.

Once we were all assembled, we sat around my father's bed, linked by his presence. The room smelled of Vaseline and the perfume of baby wipes. Dust was thick in the air. I focused on the sound of my father's breath, straining to detect any clue that would signal his course, but his breathing was regular and like a whisper.

Throughout the morning, we all remained quiet by his bedside in anticipation of the end. I looked at my watch and realized that we had already spent 2 hours in the calm of the room. My mother, who had been awake the entire night, had not yet eaten, afraid that if she left my father's side he would die without her. I wanted her to take some food, so for a moment I became a physician again and assessed my father's condition. His skin was warm. His respiration rate was thirty breaths per minute, and through a stethoscope I could hear coarse sounds from his upper airways. I listened to his heart and was amazed by its strength. The sounds were forceful, pulsing against his chest defiantly. His heart mocked the name of his illness. His heart was the real Lou Gehrig. It was the iron horse, driven to a record of consecutive days on the field.

"His heart's good," I said to my mother. "You can take a break."

"Life goes so fast," she said, distracted.

While my mother went to the backyard to eat and sit in the sun, I took her place at my father's bedside. I stayed there for almost an hour, suspended in time. His breathing was steady, almost reassuring, but when I finally looked at his face, his skin seemed more lax and his lips were mottled.

I went to get my mother. "You should go back in," I said and took her by the arm to steady her for the walk back to the sickroom.

We all came together in the living room and I announced, "It's time to say good-bye." One by one, my sister, my brother-in-law, my niece, my aunt, and I went to my father. We all cried. We all kissed him. We all said, "I love you." Because my wife and children had not made this trip, I added, "Ingrid and the kids say good-bye." For years, when I talked on the phone with my father, I would say, "Ingrid and the kids say hello," but this time the message had to change.

My mother then spoke, and with words of power and stark eloquence, she recounted their life together. I heard of joy, love, injury, regret, and a wrenching wish to stay together. "We'll meet again," she said, and her tears came again, and then she was silent.

My medical judgment was wrong. My father would not die until later that night. When I look back on that day, I think that my father rallied briefly because these were probably among the richest moments he had ever spent. His family, whom he so cherished, infused him with their love, saying things that only the deathbed would allow. These were words he would have savored throughout his life, but only in his death did he have the chance.

"This could go on all night," I said later that evening. A single lamp shone, casting a yellow-gray light on the room.

"What's the hurry?" my mother said, wistful and ironic.

I closed my eyes to the sound of the breathing as a calm descended on me and time passed without boundary. I must have fallen asleep because the next thing I can recall is my niece saying, "His breathing changed. What's wrong?"

Instantly, I awoke as I had been conditioned to do as a house officer. I looked at my watch. It was 2:00 A.M. I looked at my father. He was agonal.

Suddenly, the room became frantic with sound. I roused my mother, who had fallen asleep in a chair next to my father's bed, her hand on his.

"You'd better wake up."

"Is he dead?"

"Not yet."

"Did I miss it?"

"You didn't. He's still alive. He waited for you."

Gasp. Silence. Gasp. Silence.

Silence, and then my mother's moan, shocked, wounded, and despairing.

He was dead, and we all cried again and said good-bye once more, this time to a body whose flesh had stiffened and whose mouth now gaped.

At 6:00 A.M., two men from the funeral home removed my father's body. One had hair that was thick with pomade. The other stuttered and wore a Red Dog T-shirt visible under a white shirt of thin polyester. They wrapped my father in a sheet and drove him away in the back of an Oldsmobile station wagon. It was over.

Among the many feelings of that day that commingle in my mind—grief, sadness, guilt, longing, relief—there is also a surge of pride and even exhilaration. My family did not abandon my father at the time of his death. We did not cast him from his home and surrender him to the hospital and its fearsome machines. We kept him where he wanted to be, in a room where we had watched Ed Sullivan and Marshal Dillon, where we had celebrated graduations, marriages, and births. And just as death put my father under a spell that day, my family put death under its own spell.

Soon I will have to discuss end-of-life issues with the family of a patient who is old, near death, and defeated by illness. I will sit in a dreary alcove with pastel walls and plastic furniture. I will explain the meaning of cardiopulmonary resuscitation, intubation, cardioversion, and all of the options that are available when the heart stops, as if issues of such complexity can be distilled into a few sentences of approachable dimensions.

"What are the wishes of the family?" I will ask, as they look back and forth at each other to determine who will speak. And if anyone says, "Doctor, we want you to do everything," I know what I would like to say.

I would like to say, "Family, only you can do everything. Only you can talk of your love and give kisses before the skin is cold. Only you can talk of the future and of dreams to be fulfilled. Only you can talk of the past when life was resplendent because time seemed infinite.

"Family, only you can oppose the flow of time and enjoy one last day together. Only you can give peace and sustenance for the next journey. Family, only you can do everything. I am only a physician. I can do nothing at all."

Venus on the Right

WILLIAM G. PORTER, MD

One of the joys of our summer vacations on Nantucket is seeing our friend Eileen, now in her early 70s, who lives year-round on the island. For years, Eileen taught biology in Providence at the Quaker girls' school my wife attended. But in all her years on the mainland, her heart never left her native Nantucket. At the end of every school year, she hurried home to enjoy summer on the island. When she retired, she went back for good to her cozy house at the edge of a meadow and settled in with her dog and cat. She took a part-time job at the library and continued her vigorous support of local causes: land conservation, the science museum, island history. She loved taking us to her "secret places," little patches of forest where Eastern yellowthroats nest or rare wildflowers bloom, the best places for beach plums and blueberries.

During one of our walks, I asked Eileen how she got through the long Nantucket winters. We talked about the books she read and her other diversions, and then she said, "I like to watch the way the sun sets over my meadow every afternoon, how it moves north and south as the seasons change." Close observation of the natural world—the direction of the wind, the rise and fall of the tides, the night sky in different seasons, gave her great satisfaction.

Eileen's first extended time away from Nantucket was to attend Radcliffe on an academic scholarship. When her class held its 50th reunion last summer, she was chosen to give the keynote address, a tribute to the esteem in which her classmates hold her and to her eidetic memory for the characters and events of her college days. Perhaps she was chosen, too, because of her enduring gratitude, oft expressed, for having had the chance to attend such a fine school. Coming as she did from a small town, a working-class background, Eileen was intoxicated by the atmosphere in Boston and Cambridge—all those bright people pursuing excellence in so many fields. Including medicine. There had never been any doubt in her mind that Boston deserved its reputation as the world's premier medical city.

Eileen has a physician on Nantucket, but when she developed angina several years ago, she was quick to seek consultation from a cardiologist in Boston. Every year, she would go for an evaluation and stay for a few days with her Radcliffe roommate, Joan, a high-minded Irish Catholic spinster like herself.

Eileen came back from these annual consultations reassured that her condition was stable and, after a celebratory ice cream cone with us on her birthday, she would resume her diet and exercise regimen, a small price to pay, she often said, for the blessings of a long and happy life. "Ah, me, aren't we lucky," she liked to say, marveling at the perfection of those shared high summer days on Nantucket.

But last winter, Eileen's angina became unstable, and early one cloudless winter night she was medevaced by helicopter to a Boston hospital. Despite her pain, she was excited at the prospect of her first helicopter ride; she asked to be allowed to sit up so that she could look out of the chopper during the trip. "Nothing doing," the medic told her, so she obediently lay down on a stretcher and was borne west with the night.

Supine and restrained, Eileen could still see a patch of sky through the helicopter canopy. When she got to the hospital, her friend Joan was there to meet her. "How are you?" Joan asked.

"Oh, I still hurt a little, but I'm fine," chirped Eileen. "I had Venus on my right the whole way across."

She wasn't fine, of course. She had critical narrowing of one of her coronary arteries and was hustled off the next morning for percutanous transluminal coronary angioplasty and stent placement. The procedure went well, and an exercise test afterward confirmed a positive outcome. That was the good part.

Three days after the procedure, Eileen was discharged, according to the hospital's "standard protocol." The trouble was, Eileen's was not exactly a "standard" case. It snowed more than a foot that day in Boston, so returning to Nantucket was out of the question. Joan was happy to have Eileen come and stay with her but could not drive to get her because of the snow. As the storm intensified, Eileen's departure was delayed several hours until arrangements could be made to pay for and have delivered $400 worth of low-molecular-weight heparin (not part of the hospital's formulary) from an outside pharmacy—a transaction that caused Eileen considerable agitation because she had left Nantucket without her checkbook or credit card and had to make several telephone calls to arrange payment.

Heparin in hand, Eileen climbed into the back of a cab and was dispatched into the teeth of the blizzard with no star to navigate by. But she left the hospital without protest, secure in the knowledge that so fine a Boston hospital would not compromise her safety or the quality of her care just to avoid the expense of extending her stay another day because of the weather.

After half an hour of slipping and sliding through Boston's deserted streets, the cab delivered its exhausted fare to Joan's apartment. Eileen was so weak that she required help getting into the elevator, and when she got inside the apartment, she began to have chest pain again. Refusing Joan's offer of food and drink, she said, "I just want to lie down." Forty-five minutes later, despite three nitroglycerin pills, her pain was worse. Joan called 911, and an ambulance came and took Eileen back through the snow to the hospital's eerily empty emergency department. Soon after arrival, Eileen had a cardiac arrest, was resuscitated, and underwent urgent cardiac catheterization, which confirmed a thrombosed stent and a myocardial infarction. With good care and good fortune, she survived.

After several days of convalescence, Eileen was once again ready for discharge. Good weather made for a less arduous second trip to Joan's apartment, where she stayed for 2 weeks before going home to Nantucket.

Joan was so concerned about the way Eileen had been treated the day of the storm that she wrote the hospital. Why, she asked, had Eileen been sent out into a blizzard so soon after undergoing a major cardiac procedure? Would it not have been safer, less anxiety-provoking, to keep her in the hospital until the storm had passed? Might not such a strategy have prevented the stent thrombosis?

Three weeks later, a response came from the president of the hospital and the attending physician. After acknowledging the facts of the discharge and its aftermath, the attending physician concluded, without apology or warmth:

> She had stent thrombosis within 1 hour of arriving at (her friend's) home in Cambridge. This is an unfortunate outcome but one which was not predictable. On every regimen, there are a few patients who develop acute stent thrombosis. The current regimen, which this patient received, is the regimen which we believe gives the lowest chance of stent thrombosis.

The president added,

> I hope this [the attending physician's letter] will convince you that appropriate attention was paid to her medical care, and that the unfortunate consequence of stent thrombosis which developed shortly after her discharge and arrival at your home in Cambridge was one of those events that occasionally occur despite *the best of treatment* [italics added]. I am glad that on subsequent readmission, we were able to be of some help, and I hope that she is continuing to do well.

Yes, thank you, she is continuing to do well. But I wonder what she thinks now about the quality of medical care in Boston. Does it still deserve unqualified gratitude and respect, the way everything else in Boston does, in her scheme of things? Is she "lucky" to have been treated the way she was? Does she wonder if any hospital, anywhere, uses Venus as a navigational aid? Or does she share the nagging suspicion that whatever their histories and reputations, hospitals everywhere seem to be more influenced by the bottom line than by the taillights of a taxi receding into the blinding snow?

Conversations with Stella

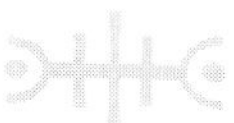

DEAN GIANAKOS, MD

Stella and I are good friends. She trusts me, I trust her. On the phone today, she tells me about her fever and cough ("Emphysema is hell"). I tell her to call the rescue squad. She tells me not to put her on a respirator ("Last November was hell"). Stella is smart and capable of making decisions for herself.

I wonder whether she really means "no" this time. One question or statement in a conversation can make all the difference. On the way to the emergency room, I imagine several different conversations.

Dr. G.: "Stella, you told me on the phone not to put you on a respirator."

Stella: "That's right."

Dr. G.: "Under no circumstances?"

Stella: "Under no circumstances."

Dr. G.: "I understand. I will respect your wishes."

Stella: "Thank you. I knew you would. You have relieved my concerns about dying helplessly on a machine."

Dr. G.: "Please let me know if you change your mind."

Stella: "I'm quite sure about this."

Dr. G.: "Stella, you told me on the phone not to put you on a respirator."

Stella: "That's right."

Dr. G.: "Under no circumstances?"

Stella: "Under no circumstances."

Dr. G.: "What if I put you on a respirator for two or three days until you recover from pneumonia?"

Stella: "Two or three days and back to my usual self? Well, that's different. I can handle that."

Dr. G.: "I understand. I will respect your wishes."

Stella: "Thank you. I trust you very much."

Dr. G.: "Stella, you told me on the phone you don't want to be put on a respirator."

Stella: "That's right."

Dr. G.: "Under no circumstances?"

Stella: "Under no circumstances."

Dr. G.: "What if I put you on a respirator for two or three days until you recover from pneumonia?"

Stella: "Two or three days and back to my usual self? Well, that's different. I can handle that."

Dr. G.: "Of course, I can't guarantee that you will recover from pneumonia."

Stella: "Forget it—don't put me on any machine."

Dr. G.: "Stella, you realize that you may die without the machine."

Stella: "I understand. I do not want to be on a breathing machine under any circumstances. I have lived a full life and do not want to risk dying helplessly and painfully on a machine."

Dr. G.: "You're the boss. No respirator."

Stella: "Thank you. I'm lucky to have a doctor like you."

Dr. G.: "Stella, you told me on the phone you don't want to be put on a respirator."

Stella: "That's right."

Dr. G.: "Under no circumstances?"

Stella: "Under no circumstances."

Dr. G.: "What if I put you on a breathing machine for two or three days until you recover from pneumonia?"

Stella: "Two or three days and back to my usual self? Well, that's different. I can handle that."

Dr. G.: "Of course, I can't guarantee that you will recover from pneumonia."

Stella: "Forget it—don't put me on any machine."

Dr. G.: "Stella, you realize that you may die without the machine."

Stella: "I understand. I do not want to be on a breathing machine under any circumstances. I have lived a full life and do not want to risk dying helplessly and painfully on a machine."

Dr. G.: "You're the boss. No respirator."

Stella: "Thank you. I'm lucky to have a doctor like you."

Dr. G.: "One more thought, Stella. Can I negotiate something with you? How about this: If you are no better after roughly three or four days, I will take you off the machine. At that time, if you are suffering in any way, I will give you medicine for comfort and relief. On the other hand, if you show signs of improvement, we'll continue support. For how long? What do you think about leaving that to me?"

Stella: "Okay. I trust you. No more than a week or two. Promise?"

Dr. G.: "Promise."

The rescue squad carries Stella through the doors of the emergency room. She struggles to breathe.

Dr. G.: "Stella, about what you said on the phone. You know, about not wanting to go on a respirator."

Stella: "What's to discuss?"

As I Was Dying: An Examination of Classic Literature and Dying

ROGER C. BONE, MD

Medical training rarely deals with helping the dying patient find peace and comfort. In fact, most physicians are uncomfortable with the entire subject. I believe it is one of the most neglected aspects of medical care. I have spent my career as a pulmonary and critical care physician, and I have cared for thousands of dying patients. In many cases, both the patients and I knew that they were dying. After I provided clinical and supportive care, I would walk away from their bedside and go on with my work and go home to my family.

Now the world has turned around for me. I have widespread metastatic disease to my lungs and bones.

When the diagnosis of metastatic disease was made, I found myself unprepared to deal with my own mortality. I tried many avenues in an attempt to come to grips with my disease. I threw myself into work and writing. I contacted old friends for solace. My friends contacted me. I discussed all possibilities of cure with many physicians across the United States and the world and chose what I believe is the most hopeful course. And, I decided to examine the classics to see how great writers dealt with death in their poetry, drama, and philosophical and fictional writings.

I was searching for peace. I hoped I might find it either in literature or in the accounts of how great writers dealt with their own mortality. But largely, literature dealt with life rather than death. No great insights appeared. Actually, the most fascinating revelation was how rarely literature does provide insight into death. One notable exception was the poetry of Emily Dickinson, who wrote frequently about death. For me, some of her most revealing lines include those below:

> After great pain, a formal feeling comes—
>
> . . . .
>
> This is the Hour of Lead—
> Remembered, if outlived,
> As Freezing persons, recollect the Snow—
> First—Chill-then Stupor—then the letting go—
>
> (#341)
>
> I've seen a Dying Eye
> Run round and round a Room—
> In search of Something—as it seemed—
> Then Cloudier become—
> And then—obscure with Fog—
> And then—be soldered down
> Without disclosing what it be
> 'Twere blessed to have seen—
>
> (#547)
>
> Because I could not stop for Death—
> He kindly stopped for me—
> The Carriage held but just Ourselves—
> And Immortality.
>
> (#712)

I found another rare exception in Louisa May Alcott's *Little Women*. The description of Beth's death is one of literature's few accounts of a character's experience at the moment of death:

> Seldom except in books do the dying utter memorable words, see visions, or depart with beatified countenances, and those who have

> sped many parting souls know that to most the end comes as naturally and simply as sleep. As Beth had hoped, the "tide went out easily," and in the dark hour before the dawn, on the bosom where she had drawn her first breath, she quietly drew her last, with no farewell but one loving look, one little sigh.
>
> With tears and prayers and tender hands, mother and sisters made her ready for the long sleep that pain would never mar again, seeing with grateful eyes the beautiful serenity that soon replaced the pathetic patience that had wrung their hearts so long, and feeling with reverent joy that to their darling death was a benignant angel, not a phantom full of dread.

The words "Please come here and help me" are uttered by Ivan Ilyich near the end of his life in Leo Tolstoy's short novel *The Death of Ivan Ilyich*. This profound work of literature is one of the greatest explorations of life and death ever written. Ivan Ilyich, an ordinary man living in late 19th century Russia, has a family, is educated, and serves as a judge. He is also faced with an incurable disease. He travels a physical and psychological path both tortuous and painful, the same path those of us who are terminally ill must face. He consistently resists asking for help, believing that by doing so, he is resisting his disease. But he eventually comes to understand that his family and friends are there to help him. Only then can he say the words "Please come here and help me."

In *As I Lay Dying*, William Faulkner writes about a woman named Addie, who is dying, and her son Cash, who is building her coffin. Addie's daughter stands by her mother, fanning her. Addie wants to be buried near relatives in another town. The novel is a parody of the distinction between being and not-being. The family is afflicted on the way by flooding, the loss of a horse that pulled the wagon, and buzzards. Faulkner makes reference to the family madness: "In sunset we fall into furious attitudes, dead gestures of dolls." Faulkner portrays the gesture of pathos of this poor family with a dead body that used to be their mother.

In Hemingway's *For Whom the Bell Tolls*, we learn that "Any man's death diminishes me," and, in his *The Old Man and the Sea*, that the virility and courage of youth extends to "old age." The latter novel was Hemingway's last and, in my opinion, finest work. The book focuses on a Cuban fisherman, Santiago, who squares off with the forces of death and emerges victorious. The reader feels that even if a man dies he can obtain a spiritual victory from the battle and emerge victorious—that life is a struggle, but the value of life lies in how we deal with it.

One of the most perceptive plays that I examined was *Our Town* by Thornton Wilder. This is a contemporary (1938) play set in a mythical small town in America, Grover's Corners, New Hampshire, about ordinary people—ordinary people who allow life to pass them by without even recognizing it. Wilder makes the point that, as human beings, we often are blind to the daily wonders of the world. He shows that life can end quickly, without warning. He shows us that we should not be caught up in the everyday rat race. In sum, his message is: Life is short: Take time to smell the roses.

In *Walden*, by Henry David Thoreau, Wilder's theme appears some 80 years earlier. "Man becomes like machines whose sole purpose is to make a living," Thoreau tells us. "The mass of men lead lives of quiet desperation." Thoreau goes to Walden Pond to search for his soul. He is seeking serenity and fulfillment. Thoreau says, "The better part of the man is soon ploughed into soil for compost. They become employed for what they call necessity, and then gather up treasures which moths and dust will eventually destroy and which thieves can break through and steal." He counsels that men should commune with nature. If he takes himself to the woods, he can learn more about himself than in the rest of the world. (One wonderful quotation attributed to Thoreau seems to show his inner peace near the time of his death. When asked "Have you made peace with God?" he humorously replied, "I didn't know we had quarreled.")

The return to Nature as Answer was also provided by Ralph Waldo Emerson in his essay "Nature." He felt that the best kind of solitude was the sort that encouraged meditation, best accomplished when man was alone with nature. Emerson believed that the soul existed before birth. He felt the spiritual world to be more important than the material world. He explained that when man's conduct was moral, he was aligned with nature and therefore with the spirit, or Godliness, which pervades nature.

In metaphysics as well, I found some answers. In *Meditations*, René Descartes searches for truth. He tells us that one should doubt all previous conclusions, accept no conclusions based only on assumptions, and subject all knowledge to the analysis of individual thought processes. According to his conclusions, any perfect being would be imperfect without existence. Therefore God must exist. Descartes thus provides an argument for the existence of God using the scientific method.

The most important controversy was the challenge offered to organized religions. After proclaiming the dogma of papal infallibility in 1870, the pope declared that evolution was untrue. The greatest challenge was to the account of creation in Genesis. If Darwin was correct, how could God's creation of the earth in 7 days be compatible with evolution? Benjamin Disraeli asked in 1864, "Is man ape or an angel?" In 1925, the debate continued with the famous Scopes Monkey Trial.

Aristotle, in his *Nicomachean Ethics*, described in the 4th century before Christ that true happiness is found in the virtuous life. He said that happiness comes from virtuous activities that result from intense intellectual pursuits. With these pursuits, man can endure hardship and sorrow and maintain virtue and dignity. He states that no one can really be happy until death.

In *The Age of Reason*, Thomas Paine attacked institutionalized religion. He attacked the Christian Church by stating, "I do not believe in the creed professed by any church I know of. My own mind is my own church." He felt the Church "appears as a human invention, set up to terrify and enslave mankind, and monopolize power and profit." He then tried to strip away the false doctrine of Christianity. He describes the Bible as hearsay, not revelation. He said that the Old Testament stories were mostly reworked ancient pagan tales. The

New Testament was not as brutal as the Old Testament but was even more absurd. Jesus was a good man who was killed because he posed a threat to greedy priests and power-hungry Romans. He stated that early Christian leaders settled by majority vote what would make up the Bible. If the vote had been different, Christian beliefs would be different.

After all of this, Paine asserts his belief in God. He says that "The Word of God is the Creation we behold and it is in this Word, which no human invention can counterfeit or alter, that God speaketh universally to man." We see God's wisdom, power, mercy, and munificence in the creation of the universe. Paine thus returns to the thesis described earlier by Descartes, that used the scientific method to conclude that God must exist. Paine simply said that he believed in his own personal revelations, not those that were transmitted by organized religion. Paine's central message was that man could find God by looking at His creations and by using reason.

The classics may at first be troubling. How could I find comfort in them? I felt, and feel, that the Bible and the church help one communicate with God—in contrast, today, to the terror found in the greed and power of the early organized religions. The church, synagogue, and Bible, in my view, are accounts that can help us find hope and comfort. The church of today exists to provide a vehicle to study God. The ministers of today are neither wealthy nor powerful. They are in the main articulate, merciful, poor persons dedicated to the concept of helping man find God.

Sydney Carton found Him. In *A Tale of Two Cities*, Charles Dickens describes a tragic romance, both timely and universal. Carton is caught up in the maelstrom of social change just before and during the French Revolution. Before he dies, he utters his famous last words, "It is a far, far better thing that I do, than I have ever done; it is a far, far better rest I go to, than I have ever known."

In summary, the great classics, the most significant works in literary history, have had a seminal effect on the behavior and attitudes of our world today, concerning themselves as they do with the issues of love, tragedy, seduction, pride, intrigue, suspense, murder, vanity, fantasy, evil, cruelty, greed, adultery, deceit, depression, fear, brutality, hypocrisy, pride, chivalry, heroism, romance, honor, loyalty, and friendship. But only rarely do they deal with an understanding of death. Notable exceptions include the works visited above, most memorably in the scene of Beth's death in *Little Women*, Emily's death in *Our Town*, and Thoreau's observations in *Walden*. I examined the classics closely for answers and was left with the conclusion that, if you have limited time, read Thoreau, Alcott, and Wilder.

At the end of my search, I felt like Thoreau as he left Walden Pond: "I left the woods for as good a reason as I went there. Perhaps it seemed to me that I had several lives to lead, and I could not spend any more time for that one."

Editor's Note: Doctor Bone, in preparing this essay, examined the following works: *The Complete Poems of Emily Dickinson, Little Women*, "On the Death of a Young Lady," *As I Lay Dying, Death of a Salesman, The Great Gatsby, A Farewell to Arms, For Whom the Bell Tolls, The Old Man and the Sea, Our Town, Walden*, "Nature," *Critique of Pure Reason, Meditations, The Origin of Species, Nicomachean Ethics, The Age of Reason, A Tale of Two Cities, The Divine Comedy, Faust, War and Peace, The Death of Ivan Ilyich, Far from the Madding Crowd, Fathers and Sons, Anna Karenina, The Prince and the Pauper, The Adventures of Tom Sawyer, A Connecticut Yankee in King Arthur's Court*, "How We Think," "Self-Reliance," *The World as Will and Idea, The Cherry Orchard, The Brothers Karamazov, Crime and Punishment, Great Expectations, Camille, The Scarlet Letter, Moby Dick, Madame Bovary, Idylls of the King, Middlemarch*, and *Silas Marner*.

That effort speaks for itself.

My Not-So-Near-Death Experience

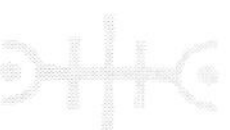

LAWRENCE N. HILL, MD

I am a hypochondriac. My medical degree offers me no immunity to this common ailment. My case is not a bad one, but I have it nonetheless. As a practicing oncologist for nearly 20 years before taking a generalist's job with the government, I empathized with my patients and became convinced regularly that I, too, had a malignant condition. Once I went so far as to walk into the reading room of my good friend, the local radiologist, and admit that I thought I might have male breast cancer, metastatic to bone, because I had discomfort in both the breast and the anterior knee. The knee films were negative, and the symptoms immediately resolved.

This time it was different. About a year ago, the fasciculations started. At first they were mainly in my calves and occurred after tennis or similar vigorous activity. At this stage, I passed them off as insignificant. But soon they began to spread, first up my legs, then into my torso and my arms, and finally to my face. Night and day, at rest and after exercise, they were there. Thirty seconds rarely elapsed without a twitch somewhere.

Oncologists don't often see amyotrophic lateral sclerosis (ALS), but the memories gleaned in medical school of twitching, bedridden patients with tracheostomies were still vivid. *Incurable. Untreatable.*

Invariably fatal. I remembered those words and phrases, but I certainly did not recall reading of any recent positive developments. I became more than a bit frightened. Previously, my thoughts of impending death had never lasted for more than a few hours, but these persisted from days to weeks to months. I was able to function; I continued to see patients and dealt with them in a professional, competent, and caring manner. Between patients, however, my thoughts turned to my own body as well as to my family and friends, who I might soon be forced to leave. I thought a lot about the physicist Steven Hawkings and figured that if I were lucky, I, too, could live a long time in a wheelchair with at least the use of a single finger. I wondered whether I could afford the special computer that allows Hawking to translate his finger movements into written and audible words.

I was living in southern Asia when the fasciculations began. I had almost no access to the recent medical literature, and the country had no highly skilled neurologists. Even if it had, I was not about to go to a neurologist. As an oncologist, I always thought it best that pancreatic cancer be diagnosed after death. In my opinion, ALS is the neurological equivalent of pancreatic cancer. I was willing to sacrifice the distinct possibility of learning that I did not have this fatal illness to avoid the equally distinct possibility of learning that I did. The anxiety of not knowing was preferable to the despair of knowing the worst.

I did have an old copy of Brain's *Neurology*. As I recall, it said something like "Most fasciculations are caused by motor neuron disease," but it also said that "Rarely do the fasciculations precede weakness." I had not had any real weakness that I had noticed, but that made me decide to test myself. I hadn't done a push-up since my Army days in 1959. I did 15 the first day, and 1 more every day for about a month. I was no Olympian, but I did well enough. Using the rheumatologist's simple test of grip strength, I inflated the bag of the sphygmomanometer to 20 and squeezed it; I moved 300 mm Hg without trying too hard. Every day I repeated this exercise, sometimes a few times—the result was always 300. I was certainly not grossly weak. Wasting occurs with ALS, especially in the hands. I spent an inordinate amount of time examining my hands. I once saw a fold in the hypothenar eminence of the left hand that I hadn't remembered being there before. I returned to the squeeze bag: Still 300, but who knows, maybe, in my case, the wasting would precede my paralyzed slide into oblivion. I tested my reflexes, looking for the hyperreflexia that accompanies motor neuron disease. Perhaps that knee jerk was a bit brisk, I would think, and maybe those hand cramps that I get when I use chopsticks aren't meaningless after all. My anterior horn cells began to dominate my thought processes.

Two or three months later, my tour of duty in southern Asia was over; several weeks of home leave in California were to precede my resettlement to southeast Asia. Obviously, California has many neurologists, including some of my old friends. I had decided not to seek an appointment with any of them. Why, I asked myself, should I have an electromyography if my outcome will in no way be affected by the results? I had also had enough experience in my medium-sized community to remember the community's response when one of its physicians developed a life-threatening illness. I had seen medical confidentiality break down in this kind of situation as often as it was maintained. I did not want to be defined by my illness; I did not want to be known as "Dr. Hill, Who Has ALS."

I did more push-ups and played lots of tennis; there was still no weakness 6 months later. I didn't have a pressure cuff, but I could still open the jelly jar when my wife couldn't. Even with these good signs, the twitching hadn't gotten any better; maybe it was a bit worse. I was pretty sure of the diagnosis. I became neither depressed nor angry. I became obsessed but, surprisingly, kept my obsession almost exclusively to myself.

Cal Ripken was about to surpass the consecutive games record of Lou Gehrig. I was on a plane between Los Angeles and Washington, D.C., and the man next to me had a copy of *USA Today*. I saw a headline about Gehrig; the subheadline alluded to a new drug for the disease that he had made famous. *The New England Journal of Medicine* or *Annals of Internal Medicine* it wasn't, but I was prepared to read anything that might give me hope. Eventually, I mustered the courage to ask my neighbor if I could just borrow the sports section for a minute. The article disappointed me; it contained nothing of clinical significance.

My usually imperturbable wife, who is well aware of my hypochondriasis, had ignored my initial undramatic lamentations, but when she saw enough of the twitching she encouraged me, both for my benefit and her own, to talk to her brother-in-law, a neurosurgeon. We did so over a beer in his television room. There was no examination. I didn't even show him my muscles. "Probably benign," he said. I wanted to feel reassured. I did, but not very.

A week later, just before my departure for southeast Asia, my wife and I were on a golfing trip in San Diego. The game wasn't too bad; my drives, always short, weren't any shorter. At the end of a round, I was told that I had an urgent telephone call from the neurosurgeon. Thinking someone in the family had died, I nervously returned the call. He said, "I talked to a neurologist friend and he is concerned. He thinks you should come in for an exam and an EMG. And by the way, does your tongue fasciculate?" He informed me that tongue fasciculations tend to be a more specific indicator of motor neuron disease than fasciculations of the trunk or extremities.

"No thanks," I said to the examination. My reasoning had not changed. The results would in no way benefit me unless they were negative, and the consequences of a positive test result were more than I felt I could handle. I hadn't given any thought to my tongue in decades, but suddenly it was the central focus of my existence. I couldn't see any obvious fasciculations in the mirror, but maybe there was an occasional flicker. Once I saw an unmistakable twitch. I felt doomed.

Why go to Asia, I asked myself, when they will only have to send me back in a few months for custodial care? Then again, maybe I'll last longer than that. Plus, I had always wanted to see Manila, Hanoi, Phnom Penh, and the other great sights of southeast Asia. And maybe, just maybe, I didn't have ALS after all. That fervent hope of a benign conclusion to the entire matter was always central to my thinking. After all, all of those other illnesses I imagined had disappeared. I went to Asia. In my work during the previous 5 years, I had departed from the United States several times. The goodbyes this time were very different. I felt strongly that many of them would be ultimate farewells, but I said that to no one.

We have a better library here in Manila than we did at my last venue. It contains the 1989 edition of Adams and Victor's *Principles of Neurology*. Continuing my amateurish attempts at denial, I waited a couple of weeks before opening it. With all due respect to those fine authors, their book's index could be better. I read the section on ALS, which reinforced the idea that it is most unusual for the fasciculations to antedate the weakness. But unusual does not mean never. I returned to the push-up and squeeze bag ritual. I was no weaker. It wasn't until another fortnight went by that I opened the text again and looked under "fasciculations." There I found the statement, "A simple clinical rule is that fasciculations in relaxed muscle are *never* (my italics) indicative of motor system disease unless there is an associated weakness, atrophy or reflex change." My response to that simple sentence was like that of a wrongly convicted man when he hears that the governor has just reexamined the evidence and spared him the electric chair.

Since then I have learned that there is a not-uncommon syndrome of widespread, continuous fasciculations that may last for months or even years. It has been described in large part in health professionals, presumably because they know about the malignant potential of muscle twitching and seek medical care accordingly. The rest of the affected population, in its ignorant bliss, thinks that they just have some twitches, not enough of a problem to warrant paying for an office call. The last line in Adams and Victor's description of the syndrome is, "Eventual recovery can be expected."

I have replayed the scenario of the past year over and over in my mind. Had I sought medical attention and had I had electromyography early on, I would have spared myself months of emotional distress. I might well have come across a sage neurologist who was fully aware of the syndrome and who could have reassured me even without the invasive test. But that would have been a gamble. On the losing side of that gamble would have been the knowledge that I had a disease that would inexorably take from me my means of movement, then my means of communication with those whom I loved, and then my life. I did not like the odds. I would probably make the same choice again today.

I'm still twitching. I don't squeeze the cuff anymore, and I've ceased doing the push-ups. I don't have Lou Gehrig disease. I am awaiting the next disorder that may cause my premature death.

Mother's Day

RONALD H. LANDS, MD

When we left home this morning, she wore a plain print dress with one of my old sweaters from college draped around her shoulders. A shiny patent leather purse, larger than a small overnight case, contained a variety of trinkets of random significance. Red Nike running shoes with Velcro snaps (necessary because she cannot tie her own shoelaces) completed the ensemble. It took me more than an hour to dress her, even after allowing her to choose the outfit.

Our separations at day care are always traumatic. She cries when I leave, and I try not to cry about leaving her. At work, I concentrate poorly because of my concerns about whether she is participating with her group and cooperating with the staff. I've had to meet once with the day care director because she was becoming disruptive during reading activities. I worry that her friends will tease her about her clothes. I dread the day when I will find, again, that she has urinated on herself without telling anyone.

She is always happy when I come to take her home. Today she was almost effusive when she saw me at the door. It gave me some hope that she may be doing better, but I can never tell for sure. Her enthusiastic smile changed to a pout when I asked her about her day.

"They wouldn't let me read to the others," she said, picking at a pair of silk summer gloves that I did not think were hers. She would say no more about it, and I didn't ask. I never push for discouraging news.

What Should I Say? Communication around Disability

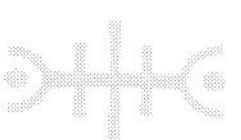

LISA I. IEZZONI, MD, MSc

Every so often, we all experience moments that crystallize an essential truth about our lives. Last spring, I had one in the cramped interstices of a federal office building in Washington, D.C. Before a meeting, I hurried to a back office to use the telephone, but a man was already there. We recognized each other instantly.

"It's been 20 years," I said. "You taught that great course on patients' experiences of illness. It helped me decide to go to medical school."

"I remember you well." He paused, eyeing me with momentarily unguarded sadness. "I heard about your troubles."

My mind raced. What troubles? Instantaneously a student again, I wondered what this professor could mean. Academic troubles? That would be too awful! Then I understood. "Oh, you mean my multiple sclerosis? I don't think of that as a trouble. I'm doing fine!"

We spoke telegraphically, catching up, until my meeting began. Later, I rolled onto the mall below the Capitol. The day was glorious, but I could think only of the encounter with my former professor. My reaction puzzled me. Why had I not immediately understood what he meant by "your troubles"? I felt that he was saddened to see me in my wheelchair; when he knew me 20 years ago, I ran everywhere. I also sensed that he wanted to hide his sorrow. This worried me; I didn't want to distress him. Why was I compelled to reassure him that I was fine? His look also conveyed admiration, something that makes me uncomfortable. Given the alternative, what could I do but go on? And, yes, what I told him was true. My MS does not feel like "trouble"—just the landscape I live in. How had I arrived at this point?

Subtexts

Although this encounter held many layers of meaning for me, one aspect is shared by all persons with visible disabilities: the implicit embargo on spoken words and the volumes of unspoken thoughts permeating our relationships with others, even our passing greetings. Communicating around disability is hard on both sides. People often don't know what to say or where to look. Silence frequently subsumes a complex tangle of fears, discomforts, and uncertainties. Other times, similarly complicated feelings prompt spoken words of many stripes: generous, tentative, hurtful, intrusive. As Sally Ann Jones, a woman with MS, said to me: "Some people see you're in a wheelchair, and immediately they raise their voice as if you are deaf. I mean, you're some kind of handicapped. They're not quite sure what to do. People aren't comfortable with handicapped people."

For those of us with disabilities, silence is often the default position. We ourselves are uncomfortable talking about our disability, concerned about breaching that invisible barrier circumscribing socially acceptable discourse. We think, generally erroneously, that silence protects our precious privacy.

But silence carries consequences. As Mrs. Jones said, "In some ways, it's your obligation to kind of educate them and make them more comfortable." Silence reinforces the stigmatization of disability, the sense of shame and guilt, and the idea that disability is something to hide. Nonetheless, opening communication around disability is difficult. What should I say? What should you say to me? One place to start is with examples of communication gone awry—what *not* to say or do. I have innumerable examples taken from my experiences and from stories told to me.

Failed Communication

Becoming Invisible

Persons in wheelchairs live below the eye level of most standing adults. Nonetheless, something other than this physical fact must make us sometimes invisible. Positioned strategically in full view of others, we often remain unnoticed. One example of this phenomenon involved a physician colleague, Megan Martin. After Megan had a complex metatarsal fracture, her orthopedist insisted that she stay off her foot for 6 weeks. I encountered Megan on her return to work, and she was frantic. Her clinical and administrative offices were far apart; on crutches, the trip had taken 45 minutes, and she was exhausted. How could she manage the multiple trips per day that were required? The solution seemed obvious. "Why don't you rent a scooter like mine?" I suggested.

As I expected—and fully understood—Megan's initial response was unenthusiastic. "People will think I'm a wimp," she worried. I did not argue; certainly they would. "I'll think I'm a wimp." That was undoubtedly true, too. In 2 days, she had rented a scooter. Later, Megan acknowledged that she couldn't have managed without the scooter, but she had remained uncomfortable and rarely left the building in it.

> [It's as if] you're not there. The few times I did take it out, it was almost impossible to get through a crosswalk before the light changed. People are crossing in front of you. I'd be sitting right at the curb, waiting to go, and somebody would walk right in front of me and then just stand there and chat for a while. Well, *they* can

run when the light changes. I thought, this is crazy. People don't want to see you; they're not going to see you.

One day after the 6 weeks had ended, Megan was standing outside my office, balanced on crutches. Nick, another physician and a nice man, approached her. "Megan, did you do something to your foot?" he asked. Nick had been around when Megan had been using the scooter. How could he not have noticed? Megan told me afterward that many people reacted the same way. They did not inquire about her injury while she used the scooter, but when she resumed the use of crutches, they asked whether she had hurt herself.

> It was amazing. It wasn't apparent what was going on until the day I was upright. And then it just hit me. Everybody knows *now*. Finally, they're noticing I've got a broken foot. Where were they all this time? It was very striking. It went from as if I wasn't there one day, and all of a sudden I'd come back after being absent for a month. The whole time it was *really* uncomfortable for people.

Seen But Not Heard

Although seen, sometimes we are not heard. For example, returning to Boston after a business trip, a colleague pushed my airport-issue wheelchair to the gate. The agent processed our tickets and addressed my colleague.

"Here's a sticker to put on her coat," the agent said, gesturing toward me with a round, red-and-white-striped sticker.

"Why?" I asked.

"It will alert the flight attendants that she needs help," the agent replied to my colleague.

"Thanks. If I need help, I'll ask for it."

"But the sticker indicates she needs assistance." My bemused colleague remained silent.

"When I need help, I'll ask for it."

"So she won't wear the sticker?"

"No, I won't."

"Why won't she?"

"Because I can ask for help."

"Why won't she wear it?"

This was going nowhere. I looked at my colleague, imploring her to stop this silliness. "Because it's demeaning," she said and rolled me away.

Not Asking

Admittedly, many people with disabilities hesitate to ask for help. We are often proudly self-sufficient and requesting assistance is hard. Sometimes we are stopped by implicitly being on the lower rung of that inevitable hierarchy of human relationships. In these instances, the right thing would be for the other person to ask us what we need, as suggested by these two examples.

A colleague, Andrea Banks, told me about one of her patients, a young man with progressive debility from cerebral palsy. He uses a wheelchair and is brought to appointments by his aunt. Andrea said that the first few times she examined him, she had him sit in his wheelchair rather than get up on the examining table. She thought that would be easier for him, but she never asked him if that was what he wanted. One day, the nurse told Andrea that the patient's aunt had complained, "Dr. Banks never even asked my nephew to walk to see how he does." The patient and his aunt were concerned that his walking had grown worse, and they wondered how Andrea could evaluate this when she had never seen him walk.

During a third-year clerkship in medical school, my MS flared up. I could no longer use the stairs when rounds with the attending physician traveled among beds scattered across several floors. As the team entered the stairwell, I went to the elevators, hoping to arrive at the next floor in time to see the team down the hallway en route to the next room. I was still in my "tough it out, don't talk about it" mode, but it nonetheless hurt that neither the attending nor the residents seemed to notice my visible difficulty in walking and left me behind. I was also timid. At that point, my attendings seemed to hold my destiny in their hands. I did not speak up until the attending paused during the closing of a fairly brutal exit interview at the end of his month.

"Didn't you notice I was having trouble walking?" I ventured.

"I did," he responded. "But because I understood you wanted to be treated just like other students, I didn't ask."

Saying Too Much

Persons with physical disabilities are frequently grabbed or touched by persons unknown and unasked. In general, this seems to be motivated by genuine efforts to help. Sometimes it preserves our physical safety, as it did when I was lifted off a busy Washington, D.C., street by several strangers after my wheelchair tipped over in a pothole. Nonetheless, unrequested physical contact can be unnerving and physically uncomfortable. Similarly, conversations can cross acceptable boundaries even if others are trying to be kind.

For example, late one evening during a third-year clerkship, I was completing my write-up at the deserted nurses' station. The new resident approached me with instructions, making it obvious that he was unaware of my situation; because of the risks posed by extreme fatigue, my neurologists refused to allow me to take call. I had asked the clerkship director to communicate this to my supervisors because I was shy and embarrassed.

When I informed the resident of my situation, he instantly responded with a barrage of questions. What neurologic tracts were involved? Was I incontinent of urine? Of stool? My legs were tremulous, and, yes, I was concerned about driving home. I answered dispassionately, as if making a clinical presentation. Apparently satisfied as to the nature of my impairment, the resident led me, virtually by the arm, out the front door of the hospital and to the taxi stand. He placed me in a cab, telling the driver to take me home and to return the next morning at 6 o'clock to bring me back. The resident then paid the driver a generous sum. Despite this somewhat surreal exchange, the resident's concern was palpable.

Suspicions

Nowadays, attitudes about so-called "entitlement" can filter down into individual encounters. The major contact that many physicians have with disability is filing forms for patients anxious to obtain dispensation from the government or employers. Physicians tell me that this often makes them suspicious of patients' motivations. Certainly, some patients do manipulate the system. However, suspicions are readily communicated nonverbally, especially to persons sensitized by embarrassment about their impairments. Judgmental disbelief is hurtful. Proving that what we experience is real can become a daunting task. As Mabel Bickford, an obese woman with bad knees who uses a wheelchair, said tearfully about talking to her physicians:

> A lot of times I don't say anything, because if things get too out of control with my doctor, then emotionally I'm drained for the rest of the day. They just think that you don't *want* to walk. You just want to be in the wheelchair; it's comfortable. Well, you try it! I'm sure this plastic cuts my legs.

Being Invalidated

A common thread of failed communication is that persons with disabilities are somehow invalidated. In the most egregious instances, the invalidation is explicit, as suggested by two examples from medical school.

One day, I encountered an attending physician, Dr. Winston, in a hospital lobby. "Hi, Lisa," he greeted me in a friendly way. "It's so good to see you."

"Hello, Dr. Winston," I smiled.

"You always seem so cheerful when I see you," he said, pausing thoughtfully. "That must be one of the benefits of the inappropriate euphoria of MS. The inconvenience of MS is compensated by you always feeling happy. That must be why you are so generally pleasant."

That was definitely a conversation stopper. What did Dr. Winston mean? Any retort would be filtered though his faulty perceptions of my mental state and thus invalidated (for example, "She's just being overemotional—it's her MS."). This encounter raised a nagging doubt: Are even my emotional stability and intellect under suspicion?

On my first day in the operating room during my surgical rotation, the attending surgeon let me hold a finger retractor during a delicate procedure. After the concentrated silence broke and closing began, the surgeon turned to me.

"What's the worst part of your disease?" he inquired.

Embarrassed by the assembled team of residents and nurses, I replied, "It's hard to talk about."

"Do you want my opinion?" he asked. The scrub nurse rolled her eyes at me empathetically. "You will make a *terrible* doctor," he continued. "You lack the most important quality in a good doctor: accessibility. You should limit yourself to pathology, radiology, or maybe anesthesiology." He turned to the anesthesiologist. "What do you think?" They planned my career.

Conversation in a Politically Correct Age

Finally, in the "politically correct" 1990s, disability has joined those topics in which language matters. Some disability advocates emphasize words, preferring, for example, "person who uses a wheelchair" to "wheelchair-bound patient." Although these preferences have solid rationales (for example, focusing on persons, not assistive devices), heightened semantic sensitivities undoubtedly chill some efforts at conversation with people who have disabilities. Our conversational partners are afraid of offending. Although I appreciate these difficulties, I believe they are quickly transcended by expressions of mutual respect and genuine interest, even if awkwardly phrased, and simple actions (for example, sitting down to be on the same eye level). As I suggest above, those of us with visible disabilities are conditioned to be "on guard."

The 1990 signing of the Americans with Disabilities Act brought the possibility that speech could convey discriminatory attitudes and presage actions that are now illegal. In retrospect, some positions expressed to me and actions taken during my 4 years in medical school (1980 to 1984) would probably be illegal under the Americans with Disabilities Act, which requires reasonable accommodations for persons with disabilities. For example, late in my third year, I began thinking about applying for an internal medicine residency. At a student dinner, I sat next to a leader at an affiliated teaching hospital, and I boldly asked his advice. I could not stay up all night, but few other accommodations seemed necessary.

"What would your hospital think of my situation?" I asked.

"Frankly," he replied in a conversational tone, "there are too many doctors in the country right now for us to worry about training handicapped physicians. If that means certain people get left by the wayside, that's too bad." There was silence around the table. During the next months, I received little support from my medical school, and after a wrenching internal debate (which was joined by my caring and realistic husband), I decided to go straight into research.

I cannot imagine that anybody would say such things now as that hospital leader did in 1983. However, although legislation can regulate actions, it cannot control thoughts. Changing pervasive societal attitudes about persons with disabilities is clearly a long-term undertaking.

So, What Should I Say?

Communication is a two-way street. Both partners control—albeit sometimes unequally—conversational directions and outcomes.

Therefore, my suggestions address persons on both sides of the issue.

For Persons with Disabilities

We should realize that many people have difficulty talking to us because of deeply embedded, complex emotions. Although overly simplistic, one explanation is certainly fear. Disability defines the one historically disadvantaged group that everyone can join in a flash. Perhaps the most obvious stigmata of disability is loss of control; this prospect terrifies Americans, who are used to being in charge. One way to forestall this horrific possibility is to invalidate those who personify it.

Persons with disabilities constantly teach others about what our lives are like and, thus, what theirs may become. I take this educational role seriously, although I try to do it by just living my life. However, although it is desirable to aim for patience in frustrating situations, total equanimity is unrealistic. Sometimes people seem oblivious to the effect of their words or actions; saying something tart and corrective may vent our irritation and improve the situation (for example, motivate someone blocking our way to move). We must contend with being dismissed: "She's just upset because she's handicapped." Nonetheless, sometimes we should lighten up. Especially in casual contacts, one cannot alter firmly rooted attitudes. We frustrate ourselves rather than change minds.

Communication with physicians deserves special mention. Persons with disabilities, especially those progressively impaired by chronic illness, must talk directly to their physicians about their functional needs. For these patients, the discussion of acute concerns often consumes clinical encounters, and functional issues remain unaddressed. Certainly, many physicians skillfully evaluate functional impairments and intercede to improve lives (for example, by prescribing physical therapy, assistive devices, or home modifications). Others, however, do not. Mrs. Jones described how her physician told her that she had MS:

> The doctor spent about a minute and a half with me, and then he said, "The bad news is, Mrs. Jones, you have MS. The good news is, when I saw you before, I wrote down three potential diagnoses in my notes. If you'd had either of the other two diagnoses, you would be dead by now." Back then, he never mentioned that to me. I said, "Why didn't you tell me?" He said, "The symptoms of the other diagnoses would have been so bad, you would've had to return, and I didn't want to upset you unnecessarily." And with that, he left. He didn't tell me what to do. He didn't say, "Do X." He didn't say, "Come back in 6 weeks." He just left. Period. He spent about 10 minutes, beginning to end. I was absolutely in shock.

Part of the problem is medical education. Many physicians know little about assessing and addressing functional problems. Until recently, most medical students were trained exclusively in inpatient settings, where acute illnesses or acute exacerbations of chronic disease are the focus. Nevertheless, another explanation is that physicians are people, too. Physicians also experience fears, discomforts, and uncertainties about confronting disability that they cannot cure. In many instances, we must educate them.

For Persons without Disabilities

My first advice is to offer us choices and options. "Do you want help?" "How can we make things better for you?" Listen, then respect our answers, even if they are a repeated "No, thank you."

My second suggestion is for you to ask yourself: "Why does talking to this person make me uncomfortable?" This need not involve prolonged soul searching. The reasons will probably be obvious; potential solutions will readily follow. For example, many people tell me that they fear saying "the wrong thing." Acknowledge this fear openly: "Look, forgive me if I say something stupid." Remember that those of us with disabilities are awkward with words, too. We are often equally anxious to ensure productive communication.

Thirdly, avoid doing what I did here—framing the argument as "us against them." I used this rhetorical device to explicate my arguments. Nonetheless, the well-worn phrase "We are all human," although trite, is true. The most visible feature that distinguishes you from me, perhaps, is my wheelchair. Each of us, however, carries private histories that differentiate us from all others; for some of us, only this one distinguishing feature is visible. For everyone, the joys and sorrows, hopes and fears that define our inner lives are invisible. Communication among people is always challenging for innumerable reasons. Identifying the role that disability plays is the first step in removing it from that complex mix of impediments.

Finally, if words and actions are obviously caring and respectful, communication will almost always be positive. For example, near the end of my first year of medical school, I was hospitalized briefly when I became completely unable to walk. Although I had tried to keep my situation secret, a classmate whom I barely knew came to my bedside one night.

"Gosh," he said reverentially, "I hear you have a really serious disease." The class had just learned about MS in neuropathophysiology.

"I guess so," I replied, uncertain what to add.

"Gosh." He paused again, obviously lost for words, but then he rallied. "I brought you a cheesecake," he said. He handed me a big box and retreated hastily. When spoken with warmth, even awkward words are wonderful.

Note: This paper was adapted from an essay that appeared in the Winter 1998 issue of *Harvard Medical Alumni Bulletin.* All proper names in this paper are pseudonyms.

Grant Support: By the Robert Wood Johnson Foundation Investigator Award in Health Policy Research.

The Examination

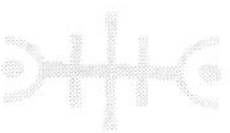

NORMAN EPSTEIN, MD

The first thing Bill noticed on that Thursday morning visit was how cool this physician's hand was. It wasn't that damp coldness some have—intimating fear and tension, no matter how reassuring the words. No, this was a mild coolness, harder to read—dry, neutral, yet shrinking the skin away slightly, a hint of discomfort. After the handshake and greeting, Bill absorbed the room's ambiance—examination areas varied from sterile to homey, and a careful look yielded a world of information. He valued any visual evidence of creativity—photographs, drawings (a sculpture would be asking too much). Any artwork was helpful, even if purchased rather than made.

Next came the examination—that was why he was here. There were a lot of issues to be raised, a lot of problems to think through, hard work ahead. The initial presentation was always the same: Bill with his symptoms—how long and where, how much and how often. Each visit had a life of its own, depending on the direction the healer needed or wanted to go. Most basic was the history—a world of information could be conveyed, clarified, implied, or revealed in the line of inquiry. Some asked little, or almost nothing, but conveyed and received so much through their other powers that it wasn't a drawback. This physician was asking his questions now, going over the chronology again, touching on the edge of Bill's dietary habits, breezing past the thick emotional and psychological forces that were woven into his body's ailments to form a chemical and spiritual tapestry. Most questions were too blunt, phrased to discourage revelation.

Then came the physical evaluation. As the physician gently probed his abdomen from side to side, Bill could feel knowledge behind the hands, but its depth, and how much wisdom lay behind it, were yet to be revealed. Bill did his own careful reading of the facial expressions and manner of touch; both men sought answers that lay deep beneath the skin, answers upon which one's universe might rotate and change. Each healer Bill had seen before had evaluated his body in a unique way, even if the training was the same, in search of a solution that would resonate, illuminate, clarify. Every examination was an adventure, an education. With this particular physician, Bill was prepared to submit to a combination of questions, physical touching, blood tests, and x-rays. He'd been through this type of examination before—it wasn't his favorite approach, but he made allowances for the orientation and philosophy of each healer seen.

Lying on the table, he focused more on the physician's breathing, changing hand temperature, inflection of voice, and body language. Bill's joints were being examined. There was a certain firmness and confidence in the physician's hands that was reassuring, as if these particular movements were more comfortable to him. It reminded Bill of an osteopath he once saw whose examination left him excited with energy and awareness well before they had finished the visit. As the physician leaned forward to look into his retina, bringing their faces almost in contact, Bill inhaled softly to gather the odors more fully—these were complex and would require sifting later, when there was time for reflection and analysis. Odors were the most difficult to analyze, and experience helped only to a limited degree. There was no retrieval of neurons lost millions of years ago, of all that lost knowledge. Bill was aware of just how primitive his olfactory sense was (a pity humans had lost so much of that useful tool).

The most delicate part of the examination for Bill was trying to sense the faint auras and bioelectromagnetic fields emanating from the healer—especially because this particular physician did not use these modalities himself. Indeed, he seemed oblivious to them. Being physically removed weakened the energy, yet touching could confuse matters by closing a contact that blurred the field and complicated it, even though the resulting combined energies were worthy of study in their own right. Healers who routinely used such energies had scanned their hands slowly above his body in a careful pattern, and he could read what he needed simultaneously. Bill remembered one who allowed him to hold his own hands over hers while she scanned and yielded to his silent questions.

While the physician wrote prescriptions and went over findings and recommendations, Bill listened intently to hear if the doctor's words conveyed consistent and coherent information. As he listened, he formulated questions in his mind. Bill always asked questions that opened wedges of doubt about the diagnosis and remedies offered—fundamental doubts rather than specific ones. After many years, he was quite proficient in asking questions that required the healer to confront the fact that many interpretations and approaches to Bill's symptoms existed. This was a critical part of the examination. A few healers rose to the challenge, looked at him thoughtfully with true curiosity and asked questions back, but he had seen many reactions, including ridicule and curt dismissal. He always looked into their eyes while they spoke.

The examination was over and the physician rose to leave. Bill always offered his hand when arriving and leaving—it was a common courtesy, of course, but was also the only time he could lay his own hands on the healer's in an acceptable way. As he shook the physician's hand, Bill asked, "Thanks so much. And how are you doing?"

"Me? Oh, fair. Just fine, thanks. I'll be calling you."

"Good. Take care of yourself."

Fair was an accurate assessment, Bill thought. He's probably in the low- or mid-B range for most areas judged, A- on overall touch (the coolness was still an issue), C in emotional intuition and receptive energies, a few areas still to sort out. This was a complex process—few were fully qualified to perform the job, but these evaluations were of tremendous value to patients and, aside from being required, were greatly appreciated. He would write his report in the morning, as usual, before going to the next healer for another examination. Never two in one day, because that made a jumble of the subtle findings and the danger of spillover was real. Like most professionals, Bill had his stories—he'd never forget the shaman he had visited in New Mexico. It had taken 2 days to write that up and a week to revert to his basal testing state so he could do another examination.

Section III

Ad Libitum

For the beginner, poetry may be approached much as one does a botanical garden. A few plants immediately catch the eye. Others might better be served as lunch to some herbivore. For some, the African violet holds a delicate beauty. For others, the flower is "too precious," over-the-top, that sort of thing. Appreciation is in the eye of the beholder, but study adds to that appreciation. Just as reading about orchids and the exacting nature of their cultivation heightens the appreciation of their rare and exquisite beauty, so does understanding the difficult construct of a sestina enable one to begin to appreciate its rare qualities.

But why bother with poetry in the first place? Why especially should busy physicians relegate their precious little reading time to the pursuit of verse? For the experience, for one reason. When metaphor, meter, tone, and feeling combine in one special poem, the experience is incomparable. Sadly, most of us physicians never know what we are missing (see *The Blossoming* by Young, p. 307)

More importantly, poetry seems to have been made for physicians, who have little or no free time and no tolerance for anyone who attempts to waste it. A nation's body of poetry is the easiest and most elegant way to understand the country's literature, customs, and thought. Poetry will teach economy: of word, of thought, of feeling, of expression. And will make you intolerant of the lack of such economy wherever you find it—In committees, for example. Joseph Brodsky has said, "The more one reads poetry, the less tolerant one becomes of any sort of verbosity, be that in political or philosophical discourse, be that in history, social studies, or the art of fiction." Someone once said that if prose consists of words in the best possible order, then poetry consists of the best possible words in the best possible order. When asked about the line between prose and poetry: Howard Nemerov wrote this:

Sparrows were feeding in a freezing drizzle
That while you watched turned into pieces of snow
Riding a gradient invisible
From silver aslant to random, white, and slow.

There came a moment that you couldn't tell.
And then they clearly flew instead of fell. (1)

How does one begin? Read through the poems contained in this section. Approach them as you would the flowers and plants in a botanical garden. Pause and enjoy those that most appeal to you. Then memorize the above poem by Nemerov. Memorize two sonnets by Edna St. Vincent Millay (2). (You can do this while commuting, if you will only shut off Audio-digest for a minute and put your mind to it.) Read two short books on how to appreciate poetry; two good ones are Stephen Dobyns' *Best Words, Best Order* and Robert Pinsky's *The Sounds of Poetry* (3,4). Then read through the selections contained in this section once again, this time choosing what you judge to be the best three poems. You can then compare your answers to those of three experts (page 362). This whole process will take you about a month in your spare time, even allowing for time for journals and for. . .television. You won't regret it.

Now allow me one bit of poetic license. To my knowledge there is only one bookstore dedicated solely to books of and about poetry.

That is Grolier's in Cambridge, Massachusetts. In this age of Walmart and Amazon.com, a store like that deserves a long life. Order your books by calling 1-800-234-POEM.

Michael A. LaCombe

References

1. **Howard Nemerov.** Trying Conclusions. Chicago and London: University of Chicago Press; 1991:101.
2. **Edna St. Vincent Millay.** Collected Sonnets. New York: Harper & Row; 1988.
3. **Stephen Dobyns.** Best Words, Best Order. New York: St. Martin's Press; 1997.
4. **Robert Pinsky**. The Sounds of Poetry. New York: Farrar, Straus and Giroux; 1998.

CONCERNING EMMA

I want to speak with you concerning Emma.
Pupils fixed, vent-dependent, she lives
as a swollen eggplant on its stem.
I understnd you gave her many joys,
sity years of prior health,
a strong voice and will, and I think
you must be very proud of her who
independently returned respect to you.
I know you are very busy and
I do not want to hold you further,
but now that I am entrusted
with her care I need your help
for though I met her only late
I must tend the leaf as best I can
and, anticipating other seasons,
turn the soil

Phillip J. Cozzi, MD

THE SHOE

Public Health Inspector
William Townsend, died 1968,
Black River, Jamaica

Townsend took a curve too fast
and died near the coast. Nobody heard
for hours. Every few minutes
I turned to the window and cursed him.
He won't come, I thought, the bastard won't.

The road from Magotty came up
a swath of banana trees battered by rain,
but the sick arrived anyway.
Glistening loudly, they filled the clinic.
We walked up and down to quiet their babies.

I was witless with anger.
Townsend had promised to come at noon
and take us away—we had such
important work to do.*Americans!*
Sister clicked her teeth at my arrogance.

At Townsend's funeral, his father
held up a shoe and cried, *He walked*
in the pathways of righteousness. I sat,
rod straight, on a folding chair
at the front of the church and didn't speak.

For isn't righteousness the brother
I never had? In Babylon,

years later, I listen for the sound
of Townsend's shoes. Playfully, he'll punch
my shoulder. I'll follow him anywhere.

Jack Coulehan, MD

NEW YEAR

The meadow that remained arid
despite last year's kisses of rain
I will make green this year,
said the cloud.

With that beautiful flower
that I did not thread in my hair last year
I will adorn myself this year,
said the garden.

That beautiful tall tree
with whom I did not dance last year
I will ask to dance this year,
said the breeze.

The New Year's crown
that I wore last year
will look much smaller than this year's crown,
said the mountain top.

The brooks
with whom I dallied last year
I will ask for their hands this year,
said the lake.

The horizon
in which I did not fly last year
will be this year's destination of my journey,
said the bird.

The dark-eyed letters
that I did not know last year
I will slip over my hand as a bracelet this year,
said the little girl.

The whirlwind
by which I was thrown back last year
I will break through this year,
said the horse.

The candles on my twelve fingers
radiate more hope this year
than last year's did,
said the candlestick on the table.

The grain of wheat
that I did not manage to store in my ant-hill
I will take there this year,
said the ant.
The poem that is shy like a deer
and that last year I could not tame
or acquaint with my eyes
I will tame this year
and take into the bright attic of my poetry-book
and let it sleep in my arms,
said finally I.

Sherko Bekas
The Secret Diary of a Rose: A Kurdish Anthology of Poems
Translated by Shirwan Mirza, MD

MY CALCULUS TEACHER MAKES A HOUSE CALL

for Lou Ulery

Why should he?
Perhaps the coach
a few teammates at the most.
But I never supposed him. After all
we both knew I had hit math's stone wall.
I was on the sofa, my right thigh
doubled-sized from a sharp knee blow
as I drove full speed for the hoop.

At the time
I think lightly on his house call
but as years pass
it becomes an act of greater weight.
So I phone and tell him
how I've come to value his kindness.
He's 83 and remembers, says
you made my day.

Still, in the right light
standing before the long mirror
I see a subtle dent across my thigh
—the scar in a fascial tear?
It's then I sometimes see him
standing at a powdered blackboard:
he's dressed in a grey suit, shirt and tie
his raised left arm keeps him oblique
to the slate, his left hand is awkward
like it's not born to write, even so
with the click of chalk he marks
delta by delta the continuum

linking x y z
while the other arm
dangles limp by his side
and the other hand
contracted into a soft claw
hangs useless
below the sleeve's white cuff.

John L. Wright, MD

TRANSFIGURATION

Underpants
lying limp, shapeless
on the bathroom floor

Shoes scattered
by ones and twos
throughout the house

Yesterday's newspaper
in disarray
over the library rug

Earrings and watch,
keys and glasses
chronically mislaid

These common objects
once grew Dragon size,
inflamed my senses

But through a gradual
Transfiguration
they have become

Small and comforting
reminders of you,
who from the beginning

Accepted
with minimal complaints
my psoriatic scales

And all other less
genetically programmed
errors.

John L. Wright, MD

THE BLOSSOMING

Genevieve
in my office, ancient, her fat chart in my hands . . .
psoriasis, arthritis, Crohn's disease, two husbands (long gone)
and now
small cell carcinoma of the lung.

"How
was the chemo?" I ask.

She has on red
high-heels, a full white dress,
a green silk scarf tied carefully around her neck,
just a hint
of perfume, and on her head
a huge straw hat with a scarlet feather . . .

to hide her baldness.

Everything
becomes clearer when I stand beside
this one flower.

George Young, MD

THE DANCING NEUROLOGIST

The dancing neurologist pleases me—
He sails the calm Aegean every Spring—
Like Sophocles, he contemplates the sea
And treats our cares as a diminished thing.
Such fancy footwork is a gracious gift—
To shift attention's locus to the feet
And let the mind's free concentration drift
To this rhythmic swaying Ionic beat.
In such a state, what relics from the past,
What precious driftwood casually afloat
Might rise to fevered consciousness at last
Or slip into the gently rocking boat?
What jealous gods or goddesses might seize
The dancing neurologist's reveries?

George N. Braman, MD

NEZ PERCÉS

I dream of Lewis and Clark
Taming the big Missouri,
Exploring a continent;
How Jefferson must have felt
When they returned, with the salt
Of the Pacific and their Indian squaw.
But the story I like best
Was of the Nez Percés, whose
Remarkable warriors went down
To St. Louis to find their old friends;
When they arrived and found
Lewis was dead, they said, "Too bad."
They never wasted words. Sometimes,
When the sunset is just right
Or a headstrong river slips away
From the voices of men, I recross
The Rockies with Lewis and Clark
And imagine I live in another
Time, a place where crags
And waterfalls are real, and paper
Grizzlies scurry from the mind.

George N. Braman, MD

"A singularity is a mathematical point at which space and time are infinitely distorted, where matter is infinitely dense . . ."

The New York Times, 12 February 1997

SUNSET ON THE TURNPIKE

Black holes and naked singularity
Keep me in constant awe of outer space—
I haven't felt the force of gravity
Collapse my inner sense of time or place.
Perhaps my limited trajectory
Protects me from the rims of galaxies
Or this confining earthbound entropy
Defies extremes of griefs or ecstasies.
Sunset on the Turnpike describes my state—
Not truly glacial, but perhaps devoid
Of cosmic movement, blending slow and late
Into a kind of twilight trapezoid—
Sky above, earth below, the sides as stark
As the event horizon, and as dark.

George N. Braman, MD

TWO OF THEM

The old Russian couple
in adjoining chairs
teeter toward each other
and tell me everything.

She demonstrates the jolt
at the edge of sleep
by jabbing a finger at me,
vindicatively.

He shows his scalp—it crawls
with emptiness at night
and keeps him up. *There,*
he bats it behind his ear.

I think he sold diamonds
for a living, enough
to convince himself, he
said once, *it's not much*
of a life. At the end
of her list is *Need sleep*
underlined twice, and *What*
happened to my eyes?

Jack Coulehan, MD

EMPTY SOUP

We made a soup last week
from turnips and thistles—
that's how poor we've become.

In the mill, our machinery
is down—we sweep the floor
all week with politics.

Better to be a free man
than a cog—stories like this
are spice for our pot.

In our lives, too—the voice
of the Russian nation
is drab and heroic

like a long family trip
after a death—so much
to do, so little time.

Empty soup—that's what
the woman from Novotny
served for her supper.

Yes, I am grateful,
she said, even for the thistles
in the cracks of my life.

Jack Coulehan, MD

STATISTICS

Between two sheets of standard deviation
She lies in her starched hospital bed.
Glancing past the window,
She reviewed the possibility
Of death at 40.

The sampling error, random, yet cruel,
Plucked her from the population.
The mass in her right ovary
Blossomed like a killing flower:
Powerful and deadly.

At night, the IV pump flashes lights,
Forcing red numbers into her veins.

Dream:
She glides down the bell-shaped curve
To the far end, to safety,
To the golden island of 5-year survivors.
Lotus eaters sip nectar (grow drowsy)
From god-smiling goblets.

Awake:
Her doctor's gaze, dry, empty.
He speaks of errors, clinical trials,
Pushing her dizzily back to the mean,
Abandoning her blessed isle.

Bonnie Salomon, MD

FOR DR. WILLIAMS*

Come round with me, Dr. Williams, in the modern
miracle hospital. Halls gleaming white:
tile, steel, porcelain.
Come round and see where we are now.
Accountants perform surgery.
Corporations deliver babies.
Billing as important as aspirin.

Come watch the technical prowess,
artificial knees, hips.
Enter frail and leave metallic.
Brave world to replace time's toll.

Visit the ER,
the portal for all troubles.
Dope addicts next to chest pain,
sore throats angry at the wait.
While nursing home patients lie
in gray stillness.
Feeding tubes supply mortgages.
The monetary supreme.

We are so lost, Dr. Williams.
The soulful touch, the faithful nod,
the peace of reassurance—
lost, hidden by fiscal reports,
tales of mergers, acquisitions,
sequestered by revenue reviews.

How to heal the wounded trust?
Examine and prescribe, Dr. Williams.

Make us whole again. Your ghost roams
these hectic halls, searching
for a quiet moment, finding poetry
where machines whir into the night.

*William Carlos Williams, MD, American poet-physician

Bonnie Salomon, MD

CHOICE

The authors (1) write that in
their study of converters three young men
were not infected by an accident
or casual carelessness. All three,
knowing well how it would be,
deliberately and with informed consent,
chose to yield themselves to HIV.

Can we believe the choice they made?
We who pray for nothing else, but pray
that we not die that way, that we evade
not only HIV, but *every* pain,
the prostate's bone-wrack or the breast's,
dementia's death in life, paralysis,
even the so-called "minor" agony
of lungs too scarred to breathe?

The reason that they gave was need to be
accepted by another, friend or lover,
already of that doomed fraternity.

For those of us who long
for the quick end, the ventricle
quivering into quick unconsciousness,
no love could be that strong,
or comprehensible,

And yet,
love has been known to do far stranger things,
when called upon to share the sufferings
of others. A myth survives that Damien
prayed once to be a leper that he might
move closer to those served at Molokai

and Catherine of Genoa when tending
the victims of another plague expressed
her love for them and for her master, Christ,
by taking purulence into a kiss.

H.J. Van Peenen

Reference

1. **Schacker T, Collier AC, Hughes J, Shea T, Corey L.** Clinical and epidemiologic features of primary HIV infection. Ann Intern Med. 1995;125:257-69.

CHEMOTHERAPY FALL-OUT

The smells of cooking greeted me as I entered the house.
I tossed a casual greeting over my shoulder as I whisked through the kitchen.
The blonde wig perched primly on the back of a nearby chair bade me glance at her again.
I paused, shocked, as she straightened from the open oven, unprepared to face her near-bald pate (hidden these months by the ever-present wig).
Disguising my dis-ease, I searched for something to say.
"I remove it when I'm cooking," she explained, "The heat singes the fibers."
"Don't wear it for me," I ventured, "It must get uncomfortable."
"Honey," she said past haunted, too-moist eyes, "I don't wear it for you."

James R. Cozzarin

BEFORE MORNING ROUNDS

No Trespassing
the haggard bit of cardboard in the puddle reads
how nice to sit so dry inside this window
on this muted grey morning
and watch as the wind
reckless outcast of ordered wards
blows rippling waves on this small lake
tossing about the cardboard raft
first this way—then that
caprice the only governing law
how comforting indeed
as dawn creeps slowly down into this space
to know there are opportunities
possibilities not predetermined
where hope can dance unfettered
and the spirit can fly with the wind

Martha Leslie, MD

GRAND ROUNDS

Women I notice that we
are by far minority
in this room full of men
with white hair
and good manners
Yet I do not feel challenged
to be more than these men are
inspired despite knowledge
of inevitable fallibility
and human fragility
the caprice of Providence
to be reckoned with
in mornings and evenings and nights
alone
gentle in passing wounded souls
who have lost the arrogance
of perceived immortality
daring a glint of laughter in the eye
spark of protection against eventuality
early light for the bonfire of hope
equally required
by men with white hair
and good manners
and challengers to fate's
harsher standards

Martha Leslie, MD

OVERNIGHT TO NEW ORLEANS

Left work at six;
by twelve, I'm in
the Café du Monde,
eating sugar-dusted beignets,
sipping coffee. Sudden
dislocations are the stuff
my dreams are made of.
They wash away
the cookpot grime
of day-to-day.

In the French Quarter,
a grungy beard, 98-proof
lists precariously
against an ornate lamppost.
Transvestites, wired, sweep by,
greeting me as if we'd just dined
al fresco on the Cajun catfish
whose aroma drifts down Iberville.
By the riverboat,
an anorectic Whole Earth Mother,
bedecked in bandannas,
tapdances on an iron grate
to streetcorner jazz.
It's much too late.
I nibble timidly: no time
to take the big bite,
even as the passersby
reel and leer
and the brutal, raucous tempos
crack my jaw.

Tomorrow, I'll dine formally
with other, starchy, suited research wonks
on haute cuisine: our randomized,
prospective, multi-institutional,
small-cell lung cancer trial,
archly debating, like wine connoisseurs,
the bouquet and color of each clause,
finetuning the fine points,
that may bring life or death
to people we've not yet met.

Corey J. Langer, MD

MEDICAL MARRIAGE

Since she had always dreamt
of making love on a beach
and he was dreaming of furrowed fields
they figured it was time

And as soon as the youngest fell off
to his nest below their bed
and the events of the day had
drifted to the corners of the room
they took the deeply planted
signs to be what they meant to be
and embraced

Later, after two more phone calls
they marvelled at their jerry-built lives
at the Rubegoldbergian blueprint
they swore once again to revise
and sang the praises of soundly sleeping children
answering machines and other small gifts
only God could have devised

Martin Kohn, PhD

IN A TRAUMA ROOM

I knew the respiratory therapist
who drew the gas
but not her name,

the name of the nurse
pushing Lasix
but nothing else.

And who was I, for that matter?
Another listener to lungs
in a Trauma Room.

"No tubes," the old man muttered
behind his oxygen mask.
"I've got no one."

At the words
we looked to each other,
before we looked at him.

Daniel C. Byrant, MD

HEALTH

By way of not defining it as an absence
Of disease or disability, let us refer
To what allows living in fullest measure.
A cardinal feature is unobtrusiveness—
No counting of stairs or hesitation
Over running for a bus. Its disappearance,
On the other hand, is sensed at once
As pain in the back or a scratchy throat
And those persistent discomforts, threatening
The knee of the inveterate walker,
The music lover's ear, the surgeon's steady hand.
More than mortality, what obtrudes is decline.

But let a man die in the fullness of his promise
And we mourn what a lost decade might achieve
Not thinking of the agonies he was spared
Or extending posthumous congratulation
On the quality his life enjoyed. Cannot disease
Harmonize living with moral overtones,
Dignity, and fortitude? And may not pain invigorate
Wellsprings of unsuspected talent, enabling
The objective expression of feeling we call art?
Perfect health, after all, might be at fault
For keeping Gray's mute Milton at the plough!

Joseph Herman, MD

THE VIRUS OF LOVE

When you seek your intended, how do you know her,
    Sweet villain,
    Bright killer?
Do you go from one to another
Looking for a lover
    One ready to receive your sting
    As if a prized and desired offering?

More important to me, who would understand love,
    Your thrust
    Does move
Your being to perfect ecstasy,
Your lover to copy
    Part of you to create new life,
    As portions of a man by a willing wife;

How can I be sure that you lack love's desire?
    You choose,
    You sire
Upon the body of another,
Oblige her to mother
    Yourself in shape of progeny
    Who assure your form of immortality;

About your mate I can be more confident,
    She dies,
    Is rent
Liberating the new life you made,
She is wholly consumed,
    Unlike our kind whose women enjoy
    Observing youth, and themselves, in girl or boy;

Among our own kind I know that some must love
  Like you,
  Who live
By compelling another to give
  The substance of her life
  As a sacrifice for him to use
For his own enterprise, as does the virus;

But whether for you or one of my own kind,
  For love,
  To have
Its power, one must stoop to receive,
The other know that she
  Is chosen by fate to receive him,
  And offer the place he seeks to enter in.

Fredric L. Coe, MD

THE CRACKING OF THE MOLD

We have known the insolent look
of the breaker of cities, the night
flying worm of the rose, the rotted
fleshy bed where it lights;
it comes to reclaim an old right,
lost to it for the brief term
that begins in the dark collusive urn,

at the beginning of the first fable,
and ends when flesh wears out
like an old butterfly, unable
to eat, lacking guts and throat,
frayed like an old coat
we fought to repair, my dear,
when our blood drummed with the fury of war.

And now your chaste hot vows,
your high and soldierly passions
are gone; two aging clowns
march to a cracked drum
and nickelodeon
before an empty stand,
hearing applause, and a marching band;

ours is an insolence
that would have us wear
these uniforms of office and defense,
like a woman, long past those years,
might pin a flower in her hair,
and dress in a girl's dress
her burned-out shell of fertileness.

What is it, then, we may take
from so long a time, so long
and disciplined a life, for whose sake
we gave much youth? It is wrong
to forget, it is as wrong
to dwell on what has gone,
and wrong to think it leaves no stain,

no print, no embossment,
"There," you say, "is the difficulty;
to bear past imprint
yet be free; for we are not free
of it, we wear the history
of war like an old bone
the marks of a dance; we are shaped by what's gone,

that visage cannot be altered
or erased, except we lose
parts of us in the endeavor."
Keep it, then, I shall choose
the same; wear it like an old jewel,
from another and a lost age,
chased with mysterious images.

Fredric L. Coe, MD

RE-CARNATION

When we reach the winter of us all
Frail Flowers
End our uneasy season
On this sun-spot
When we are ground—back to stardust
Gritty Flour
Baked in the oven of forever
Shall we all rise—spring again?
Next time.

David R. Scott, MD

NIGHT SHIFT

In the ER tonight
Another gunned addict,
Pupils blown as hubcaps,
One small hole carefully shot
Square into visual cortex.
No exit wound, but bullet raised
A tumor over the temple,
Bluish as a ripened cervix,
Brains exploded into brains.
A bored student bags breath
Down the graceful, bruised larynx
Into cold, black lungs;
A thick rope of gold rises,
Falls, slips tighter around the neck.
We track his blood across the room.

Driving home beat,
The trees sway in seizures.
Skin-headed children
Lean out of windows,
Droplets of black blood
Gashed from tenements.
Fat church-women wriggle
Festooned butts and holy arms,
Winos jive and stamp.
Infants numb from crying
And mothers without tears
Bleed into the pointblank streets.
From the dingy rooms of bars,
Needled pimps and razored whores,
Virus-wasted youth and addicts

Hemorrhage into morning
From dark alleyways.

The moon is dead,
The assassinating sun rises
Quiet, without a gleam of amazement.

Tom Di Salvo, MD

A NAVAJO SABBATICAL

When I first came
to the Navajo reservation
I was afraid of heights
I was afraid of horses running free
I could not walk the canyon rim
(too much flatland in my past).

But now I like to dance
if only
back here in the midwest
if only
before clinic in the morning.

And now I remember
when I look at the moon
a Navajo man who lived
by Coalmine Canyon
and rode his horse every day
across the high desert.

And now I hear
his high voice singing
when the geese rise
from the pond by the hospital.

And now I recall
climbing Castle Rock to the very top.

I gave the Navajos
only some doctoring
but they gave me new rest

new courage
new strength
and a poem to remember
by an unknown Navajo poet:

"Today we are blessed with a beautiful baby.
May his feet be to the east
May his right hand be to the south
May his head be to the west
May his left hand be to the north.
May he walk and dwell on mother earth peacefully.
May he be blessed with assorted soft valued goods.
May he be blessed with precious variegated stones.
May he be blessed with fat sheep in variation.

I ask these blessings with reverence and holiness
May mother, the earth, the sky, the sun, the moon together
my father
May the essence of life be old age.
May the source of happiness be beauty.
All in peace, all in beauty,
all in harmony
all in happiness."

David Schiedermayer, MD

WHAT NURSES DO: THE MARRIAGE OF SUFFERING AND HEALING

Jane Ball, Retired Nursing Supervisor

Compared to the day I had to sit with a mother
Ask for her daughter's three-year-old kidneys,
Eyes, liver, and heart because a drunken
Teenager had killed her brain
Compared to the afternoon I told a black man
His son was shot while jogging
Compared to the night I was paged to ER
To help sedate a seven-year-old girl
Before they sewed her crotch
Being here with this schoolteacher holding
Her husband's hand, begging him to live
Is better.

The rhythm of a heart repeats itself like vows
In a chapel full of light, but we are gathered
Here because this man's heart choked after forty years
Medics shocked him, brought him back
Then, a cardiologist with his pacemaker, a respirator
We have stolen these minutes
But our bag has no more tricks, no more drugs
Or gizmos, and now, something as old as love
Must be the pencil that helps the heart write
Its good-byes across our screen.

I will never forget the wife's brown hair
And her tan corduroy blazer, how her face looked
When she asked for her husband's baptism
We couldn't reach a priest. It happens.
They all looked at me: the nursing supervisor.

I said I could.
In the presence of this company
Who gives this man to the next world?
The paper cup was blue, I asked a blessing
For the tap water and did it, water fell
Soft as a kiss to his forehead.

And so I kept the devil faraway
And let the wife cry into my shoulder
For a long time after
For a long time after.

Jeanne Bryner, RN, BA, CEN

IN MARCH

I

In the chill early evening
cars dodge potholes and frost heaves
dragging their tails home
behind burnt-out headlights
in March.

House pets do the in and out dance
at the doors, after all day asleep.
Stones sit submerged in newly heated holes.
They melt craters in the blank face of mud
over everything—
in March.

Rime ice releases its crystalline clutch.
Feet sound like molars pulled out of a jaw.
Angular shards yield to the roundness of footprints.
Boots meet earth in a sloppy kiss,
and walking becomes a compensatory ice polka.

Trees shed joints, arms, bark
eased away by emerging calyx.
Pushing and shoving makes its own music
in March.

New again
Old still

hard soft
March.

II

We drive together in your cosy car cocoon
through this rich violent nightscape
to see the pale beams of the lighthouse
finger the fog.
Five streams of light flow out to the sea
answered by the gutteral groans of foghorns
at the bay's entrance.

I turn to you, vibrating with the struggle
between light and dark
winter and spring
beginning and ending
love and loss
in March—

To find you standing in silence
bewitched by the light cast so gatheringly
over the noisy sea.

We hold the brightness between us
on our way home,
to curl toward one another
in the warm dry bed.

My fingers sing songs of spring over your back.
The peace of beginning
settles over us.
The sharp anxiousness of new
melts like the wet ice outside.

I love loving you
in this now, this new,
in March.

Walden S. Morton

OLD AGE

My grandfather tells me
You may come at any time.

That you are from faraway
Staying at one place for varying times
Until the next earthquake or flood
Or till the angels call you away.

My grandfather tells me
Pretenders will falsely represent you
Complaining of fatigue, pain, boredom:
Loose changes falling out of the pocket
  of time.

That you are unpredictable
Wearing a thousand faces
Of overlapping shadows and clarity:
Icy and generous,
With periods of long soliloquies
And short temper, doubtful and foolish,
With nostalgic lapses and moments
Of capriciousness, humorous and annoying.
You are strange, sublime, caring.
Original, often misunderstood.

Shall I loiter at doctors' waiting rooms?
Shall I search my room,
Look at mirrors, the moon
For hints of your coming?

Slowly, I will prepare
The wheels of renewal:
I will eat pumpkin seeds, honey,
Wheat grains. In the desert, I
Will seek the hermits. Around my ankles,
I will chain stones and drag myself.

I will visit art galleries; listen
To Mozart, Chuck Mangione, Streisand;
Commune with Thoreau, Rilke, Pascal.

In my garden, I will grow herbs
And spices. In the darkness,
I will try to distinguish texture
And form, subtle shifts of temperature
And weights, of pebbles, furnitures,
Petals, and the different corners of my knuckles.

Because the quotient of all these works
Is a circle of wishes:
To outrun, outwit,
                outlove you.

And when you come
Bearing gifts from your ancestors:
Serenity, wisdom, forgiveness
You will not be a stranger.
I will open my doors to you
A friend meeting a friend.

We can share evenings when stars
Descend with fullness of intimate hours;

Savor the promise of each precious
Moment at San Francisco Bay.

You can teach me teachings
 of experience:
"To accept the commitments of life
By suffering, loving, bearing
Life's indignities with dignity."

I will listen to your songs
Of hundred variations of one truth.
I will watch soothing fingers of your voice
Stroke each string of my guitar.
When the air splits gossamer notes
Riding the balance of thirteen strings
I will close my eyes
 and dream.

Edgar A. Calvelo, MD

MY AMBITION

With whom are you
Flirting now, my sweet ambition? With what
Younger student are you
Nuzzling in the library stacks or melding futures
In Erlenmeyer flasks?

You ultimately grew bored
With me and, true, I was no match for you,
Full-lipped, provocative,
Tireless. And now that my latest partner has left
I can't stop thinking of you.

Did I leave you?
Or did you leave me? Uncertainty cluttered our lab
Like an incomplete experiment
Either lacking the power to answer the question
Or flawed in design.

You wanted more from me
But I wanted children and I wanted time.
You wanted perfection
Because that's what you do best: want and want
Again, satisfied never.

You wanted Hippocrates,
Leonardo da Vinci, Sir William Osler. Instead,
You found yourself flirting
With a commoner. Remember when you gave my daughter
The astronomy flashlight.

All the world flashed

On the ceiling in the dark. She has stopped
Asking for you, but
Your sweet touch of foreignness glazes her eyes
And frightens me.

Today, I see patients,
Write only in charts and taxi the children back
And forth to the library,
Glancing occasionally in my rear view mirror,
Wondering if you're there.

Phillip J. Cozzi, MD

CEMETERY AT TERLINGUA

Here in this parched and rocky ground there lie
Beside the road in closely clustered mounds
The remnants of the humble men who toiled
Their lives away in mines among the hills—
In blankets or in wooden caskets laid
To rest beneath rude crosses painted white,
But now, in scarcely fourscore years or less,
All broken, weathered, and bereft of names.
Time was when tears moistened this arid earth
As loving hands prepared each shallow grave
And placed upon the fresh-turned heaps of soil
Some small, frail symbol of eternity.

Oh, traveler, lift your eyes upon the vast
And desert scene about this tiny plot.
Behold the lava flows of long ago,
The beds of ancient seas and verdant swamps
Where lie the shells and bones, now turned to stone,
Of creatures that inhabited this land.
Behold the flow of half a billion years,
A fraction of our planet's place in Time.
Then look again upon these crumbling works
Of lowly men, and hasten to recall
That even the works of mighty kings decline,
That palaces and pyramids decay.

Small wonder then that in the loneliness
Of this infinity of Time and Space
Sentient and thinking beings like ourselves
Should crave some mooring for our storm-tossed lives.
Our human bonds we need to comfort us,

But these are often fragile and may break.
Likewise our cultures tend to change with time.
Most men, therefore, do seem to need some faith
In an uplifting power, which does not change,
To stabilize and sanctify their lives.
Hence these rude crosses in the desert thrust
To tell us there is life beyond our dust.

James E. Kreisle Sr., MD

IMG (INTERNATIONAL MEDICAL GRADUATE)

In Madras, threadworms crawl out at night
on hospital sheets glazed dun with washing.
They wriggle in the middle
of rumpled starch-stained cotton,
barely visible punctuations
to unread chapters of overwritten lives.

Morning light discovers old men furled
fever-heated, anopheles-shivered,
in bedless pockets of a gorged ward;
dreaming a womb's caress of the cold stone floor,
warmed by thoughts of noon
and the trays with lentil soup.

At three in the humid afternoon,
the Injection O.P. is full. A curving brown ribbon
twirls out its double doors;
goose-stepped rows of nude upper arms,
sacrificial lambs bereft of all fat,
awaiting the painful benediction of vitamin stabs.

Mycotic ulcers soothe with the sundown
Indian Ocean breaths, that sough soft
as mother's kiss on abraded knee,
through British-built hallways, over parallax pallets.
Families knot, around beds hard with waiting;
Tiffin carriers packed with*rasam*-rice and hope.

White coat over *sari*, nine p.m. rounds;
she brands his chest with her stethoscope
—endpiece warmed with her breath,

to thaw cold lungs, condemned to death
by mycobacter.
Her Tamil is stilted,
the mother tongue stumbles,
unable to grant a stay of execution.

Her patient coughs blood; in between hacks
he mocks her accent,
convent-English wrought.
She smiles touching him, what she lacks
in language, translated through her hand—
You are my fellow man.

II

In Los Angeles, sunsets dim from yellowbrown veils
that hang heavy over mountaintops
and festoon arterial walls
of good and bad guys alike.
Rayon-suited businessmen too rushed for life,
lend Hollywood adjectives to myocardial infarcts.

Van Gogh irises bloom on dawn-painted walls
of equipment-rich hospitals—
and wither in the eyes of anorexic angels.
Across, in the mall, the stores are thronged
with birds of paradise in apparent full bloom—
dying slow inside from the need to belong.

Pacific sun laves afternoon gold—
and melanomas—on Caucasian skin.
The beaches are full. From under the piers
young men are ambulanced, heroin cramped.

She puts away *Parasitology: A Textbook,* by Chatterjee;
searches for needle tracks on arms without veins.

Mrs. Smith at the nursing home begs her to stay,
meet her grown children—visiting hour is here.
They rock in the lobby, few families near;
Far off, a bell knells, no offspring today.
Mrs. Smith takes a long time to sleep that night.
She wishes she had brought a tiffin carrier.

White coat over skirt, night E.R. call;
The bag lady mutters, empty space
where her front teeth should be;
points to her legs. The patient sees
double—progress note from a year before.
Her English is clipped,
the second language trips,
hesitant to voice fears of multiple sclerosis.

"Garn" says the bag lady, her hisses
loud for the E.R. to hear,
"You ain't nevah hearda charley horses?"
She smiles touching her, what she misses
in idiom, translated through her hand—
You are my fellow man.

Bhuvana Chandra, MD

FRECKLES

I noticed the freckles on your shoulders this afternoon,
as a black plastic bag was pulled from your arm.
And I stood in awe of things bigger than myself as I gripped the
    table for support,
occasionally remembering to breathe.

In anticipation of this day, we made some decisions.
You, to teach
and I, to be taught.
Here we are, together now, in a marriage of circumstance.
Your body the classroom.
I, your strange new pupil, fumbling with parts of you that few,
    if any, of your closest friends ever saw.

Finally face to face,
what do you see when you look at me now?
Am I what you thought I'd be?
Eager? Anxious? Do I look as tired as I suddenly feel?
Can you see the lump that rises in my throat
as I struggle to fix my eyes anywhere but on your face
where what you once were looms largest?
Can you see the tears that fill my eyes as I grieve the loss of
    someone I've never met and
struggle for composure in a room full of people I hardly know?

You did not choose me,
yet you trusted me.
And I will never know you,
although somewhere, a family mourns the passing of one they love.

I need time, that's all.
Time to think about what this means for both of us.
Brother,
Son,
Father,
Husband,
Neighbor,
Cadaver.

I noticed the freckles on your shoulders this afternoon.
Tonight I noticed the freckles on my own.
We're the same, you and I,
only you've been There,
and I haven't.

Jennifer Best

THE FALL

Lie still, bird
with a broken wing.

Stop shivering
under the snow of your winter,
this clean white sheet.

Your hollow
bones are better for flying
than tottering down
the lonely halls of a nursing home
in ragged
bathrobe and slippers . . .

where you fell.

Now
there's a magenta bruise
in your side,
and the little blue rivers
in the glass-like skin of your temple
have spilled blood
in the white feathers of your hair.

The nurse will bring
some morphine for your pain.
And tomorrow
the orthopedic surgeon
will fix your hip with a pin.

You won't fly.
But you'll walk again.

George Young, MD

TOBACCO TAX

"Their bodies fill a crumbling room with light"—Allen Tate

The ultimate burley tariff came due
that dark-fired afternoon
when many would have paid
on his behalf if coins would clear his debt.
Yet, lungs aged thirty years beyond
the hand which had held his cigarettes
demanded currency stronger than that
as pneumonia red-penciled
his life's works like first drafts.

Around his hospital bed that night
stood boys in white, unsure, ascending,
starched, fervent, answering their pages
full of hope and healing, reading
one last biting essay from the sage
who taught a lesson in dyspnea as he died
in that spare classroom where he forgot
the first lines of his own poems,
breathing the common air.

Eric L. Dyer, MD

THE GATE

This morning I plant irises, cultivate
woolly thyme, creeping geranium, while

you give out your last breaths. Henry
said you sleep sitting up as your lungs fill.

And can't sleep. Maybe now you wish
for the end, a steady state of sleep

without hunger for air. No one
can feed you, no one can press their

fleshy fingers, cuplike, over your open
mouth, stifle the fierce fight that
brought you to the gate, not knowing
a gate was there. You said this is life

as long as you call it life and would not
let your friends murmur that other word

in their easy sleeping, those who knew
they'd wake up in the morning, weed

in the bright overgrown garden,
the sunny place where you are not.

Alice Jones

UNTITLED

If that was the autumn of her years
This would be the winter
For then her leaves were turning
A scent of coolness in the air
Was a reminder of other autumns we have known
When songbirds had taken flight and flowers closed
The warmth and sparkle of summer's air
Had faded into memory
And cool and misty breezes blown

But now her leaves have fallen
Her branches stand exposed, her graces lost
The colors of maples, birch, and marigolds
The bounties of the harvest
Have been replaced by snow and frost

Do we look with memory's eyes
And long for summer's warmth
Or recall the joy of spring
And grasp the memories
Which for her have fallen like the leaves?
I try not to see
A desolation in her eyes
A north wind drifting snow
Across a prairie or a frozen bay
In this starkness
Let me think that she is unencumbered

J. Kelly McGuire, MD

A LIGHT LAMENTATION

Now Newton thought he'd got it right
when he described the waves of light.
Then Einstein said, "Oh no, I want a
have you think of light as quanta."
And Schrödinger suggested that
a single one could kill a cat.
Now that's too much for me, I'm scootin
back to the waves of Isaac Newton.

Grant Gwinup, MD
Dayna Diven, MD

KOREAN SKETCHES: THE LEPERS OF PUSAN

We moved in
Spearhead of mercy, caduceus-clad
Hope sewn into our arm bands
Red on white spangling our vehicles
Like vulgar billboards

The advanced party, serious
Horn-rimmed with stacatto pencils
Racing over creased notebooks
Fingers convulsing the iris of cameras
Toward every door

And they
Sullen in their private anguish
Half men and part women
Staying the pallid children
With their almost hands
Frozen like rabbits in the brush
Awaiting the advance of these strangers
Measuring the hunter through blistered eyes
Leonine faces telling nothing
But the obscenity of their misfortune

We split open our cartons
In the clay-baked square
Under a cloud of flies
Heaping our offerings
On trembling tables
And stood in smiling ignorance

Soldiers of the Christian world
Waiting for these banished brethren
To recognize the love of man
Incarnate in cigarettes and chewing gum

Alvin L. Ureles, MD

THE PALINDROME

Ignaz Semmelweis,
who cut the maternal death rate
in the *Allgemeines Krankenhaus*
obstetrical ward
from 18 to 1.2 percent
by insisting that the doctors
wash their hands
before and after
each exam and delivery,
so outraged his colleagues
by his findings
that they hounded him
back to Budapest
where he wrote
Die Aetiology der Begriff
und die Prophylaxis des Kindbedfiebers
and, in 1865, died of sepsis
in an insane asylum,
a brokenman.

In Brockelman's Market,
a woman, pregnant,
her blouse a color
between faded yellow
and yellowed white,
between spit-up milk
and rebleached diapers,
a tired woman who, soon,
for the sixth time, won't
die of childbed fever,

is buying warm
whiterolls.

Paula Tatarunis, MD

POETRY PRIZE WINNERS

If you read the introductory piece to the "Ad Libitum" section, you will be looking here for the best poems of the last three years as selected by skilled practitioners in the field.

In 1995 the Board of Regents of the American College of Physicians (now the American College of Physicians–American Society of Internal Medicine) initiated an annual Poetry Prize of $500 to be given to the author of the best poem published in *Annals of Internal Medicine* during any given calendar year. The judges have been three nationally known poets:

- John Stone, whose most recent book of poems is *Where Water Begins*, Louisiana State University Press, Baton Rouge, 1998
- Donald Hall, Poet Laureate of New Hampshire and man of letters, whose most recent collection is *Without*, Houghton Mifflin, Boston, 1998
- Daniel Bosch, instructor in creative writing at Harvard and winner of the first annual poetry prize from *The Boston Review*

The first three winners of the *Annals of Internal Medicine* Poetry Prize are:

1996 - Phillip J. Cozzi, for *Concerning Emma* (page 298)
1997 - Jack Coulehan, for *The Shoe* (page 299)
1998 - Paula Tatarunis, for *The Palindrome* (page 360)

Did your selections match those of the experts?

Michael A. LaCombe

About the Editor

Michael A. LaCombe, a graduate of Harvard Medical School, has developed a career that blends writing with over 20 years of medical practice in rural Maine. He has written several books (*Medicine Made Clear: House Calls from a Maine Country Doctor*, Dirigo Press, 1989; *The Pocket Doctor*, Andrews McMeel, 1996; *The Pocket Pediatrician*, Andrews McMeel, 1997) and has edited and contributed to *On Being a Doctor*, American College of Physicians, 1994.

Doctor LaCombe is editor of the "On Being a Doctor" and "Ad Libitum" sections of the *Annals of Internal Medicine* and has edited the "Medicine, Science, and Society" and "Reading for Survival" sections of the *American Journal of Medicine*. More than 80 of his stories and essays have appeared in publications such as the *Journal of the American Medical Association*, *American Journal of Medicine*, and *Hospital Practice*.

Public readings of his short stories have been given by Dr. LaCombe across the United States and internationally. He has served as visiting professor of medicine at over 40 medical schools and university hospitals, including Yale, Harvard, and the University of California at Los Angeles.